OF

MONKEYS

AND

DRAGONS

OF
MONKEYS
AND
DRAGONS

Freedom
from the
Tyranny of Disease

By Michele Longo O'Donnell

LA VIDA PRESS

SAN ANTONIO

First Printing 2000
Second Printing 2002

Copyright © 2000, 2002
by Michele Longo O'Donnell

Library of Congress Card Number:
00-105945

ISBN: 0-9676861-0-5 (HARD COVER)
ISBN: 0-9676861-1-3 (TRADE PAPER)

Published in 2000 by
La Vida Press
410 West Craig
San Antonio, Texas 78212
888-493-8660

Printed in USA

Cover Illustration by Travis Ward

TO PEGGY AND RAY

AND ALL WHO HAVE SUFFERED THE
RAVAGES OF DISEASE.
MAY WE COME TO KNOW
HOW NEEDLESS IT IS.

Write the vision and engrave it so plainly upon tablets that everyone who passes by may be able to read it easily and quickly as he hastens by. For the vision is yet for an appointed time and it hastens to the fulfillment: it will not deceive or disappoint.

Wait earnestly for it, because it will not be behind on its appointed day.

HABAKKUK

LETTER TO THE READERS:

It has been eighteen months since this book was published and after hearing from hundreds of readers, I thought it prudent to add this addendum to the second printing.

Since its first appearance, we have had the book translated into Spanish for those folks who are more comfortable in that language. I have had the opportunity to hear back from some of my patients from Mexico, and all points south, and they are sincerely appreciative of our effort in getting the book translated into their native language. We also have made the book available on CD audio for those who, for whatever reason, would enjoy hearing me read the book to them.

Another addition since the original printing are my weekly radio shows originating from San Antonio, Texas, called, "Living Beyond Disease." From these broadcasts we have developed an extensive list of "teaching tapes" which have proved to be extremely beneficial in enabling our readers to implement these basic principles of health and living. Please check our web site for availability. (www.micheleodonnell.com)

I have been traveling all over the country speaking and sharing these truths to "hungry hearts and thirsting souls". I have been blessed with such an outpouring of sincerity, as I could never describe. But the most wonderful experience of the past year or so has been those who write or call describing healings that they have received after reading the book, attending one of the lectures or listening to the tapes. There truly is a River Of Life that flows around and about us, with healing in its waters, available to all and anyone who wishes to experience it. It is a Spiritual Flow of Divine Life and in moments of silence one can hear it calling to us, saying, "Whosoever will, let him come". "Whosoever thirsteth, let him drink".

Gone are the days where we believed we had to earn such an experience, or "qualify" by some man made standards. Gone are the days when God was so far from our reach, when we felt so lost and alone and forsaken. Never has the Spirit of God come so near to men's hearts as It is now. While we appreciate the efforts of the clergy and doctors and various healers available, this is about you and your Creator, you and the heart and mind of Eternal Love. He is as near as the breath you breathe...you walk and talk, live, love and laugh within the substance of this infinite and holy Life. It contains all that you need now or could ever imagine yourself to need. It will be your teacher, your guide, and your friend. It will show you the face of God in everything that you look upon. It will purify your heart and emotions, TEACHING YOU TO LOVE, in the face of the most abusive and obtrusive circumstances. It will correct and show you the way in every situation.

My greatest joy is your life restored and made whole. As the veil of this convoluted and confused world and religious views and beliefs are lifted from you, you will enter into the glory of your "first estate," which is that infinite and present perfection of the image of God, the wholeness and holiness of Divine Life. Everything then will appear new. "The earth is the Lord's and the fullness thereof and all them that dwell therein." Held deep in the Mind that is God, "the works were already finished from before the foundation of the world." You will find that what you seek after, you have always and already posses. Don't let anything that you see tell you differently. Don't let anything you hear tell you differently!

My love to every honest seeker,
Michele Longo O'Donnell

CONTENTS

ACKNOWLEDGMENTS

To Linda and Lara—my best reason for living and the reason I pressed on.

To George—a kinder and gentler man never lived. Thank you for your patience and support.

To Carol and Julene—thank you for your encouragement and infectious enthusiasm.

To Nancy—my mentor, my teacher and my friend. Thank you for the many years of patience and endurance. Thank you for your faithfulness to your calling and to me.

To Melissa—my dearest friend, without whom this work could have never happened. Thank you for taking over my responsibilities at the clinic, to free me up so that I could write. Thank you for your heart of gold, for your love for the work, your love for the patients and your love for me.

PREFACE

My lifelong goal has been to find a way to end the tragedy of suffering by disease. I always felt that it was an *intrusion* in our lives, never a necessity. Therefore I believed that there was a solution.

At first I was somewhat content to *take care* of those who were sick. Just deal with individual diseases and cases as they appeared. Find a solution for each one, another pill, another program. But as the years progressed, I realized that there was no end to it all. New diseases, new names, new descriptions and new symptoms would appear on the horizon of human experience in direct proportion to the extent of human imagination. If we can imagine it at all, we can experience it. So in frustration, I turned my weary footsteps away from a path that I knew would never end. And I began to look for the source of it all.

As the journey progressed, I found that the same cause of suffering from disorder in the body was true of all human pain and anguish, regardless of its appearance. I saw all the present efforts toward the relief of human suffering somewhat like frantically swatting at flies, but leaving the pile of garbage that was drawing the flies unnoticed. The futility of our efforts at the present level of medical, and even alternative care, is staggering.

Instead of more million-dollar machinery, instead of more surgical procedures, instead of more pills with more toxic side effects, instead of more insurance, instead of more alternative cares cropping up . . . we need answers.

The task was, and is, formidable. And I am, more than anyone else, aware that no individual human being is up to such a task. But I do believe in the ever-presence of God, as the Divine Intelligence, Who set the whole scenario in order, and Who continually communicates with us, if we would only learn to listen. That, I believe, is the only place that we will ever find our answers.

I am aware that the subject written about in this book will be met with both joy and criticism alike. It would be impossible to explore such a delicate topic, fraught with so much emotion, without liberating some and infuriating others. While my intention is never to incite negativity, still my desire is so strong to see those suffering freed from their slavery to *belief* in disease, that I am willing to "duck the blows" in order to gain the goal.

Please remember throughout your reading that I am

relating a mental and emotional and spiritual journey of my own. My deepest emotions, my strongest desires are poured out on these pages. The events that are shared are real and interpreted according to my personal journey toward spiritual understanding in the question of human suffering.

Realizing that people come from multitudes of individual backgrounds of thought and beliefs, and rather than try to satisfy the integrity of each one, I did the only thing left to me to do, which was to tell it as it unfolded to me and pray that it will reach the hearts of those to whom it was intended. So, if you come to a bump in the road as you are reading along, and you probably will, try to just hop over it and go on. Hopefully, it will all *come together* for you in the end.

INTRODUCTION

Generally authors develop an introduction which declares why they are qualified to know and to write the material which is presented. They give details of their accomplishments and achievements, which are intended to lend credibility to their words. After much thought and struggle over such a task, I have decided to tell you instead, why I do not qualify according to human standards, to know what I know, to understand what I understand and to do what I have done.

At seventeen years of age I entered a nursing school program by the grace of God and the kindness of a Catholic nun/ director of the school of nursing. I say, by the grace of God, because academically I didn't meet the standards for entrance into this discipline, not having completed chemistry in high school. But for a reason beyond my understanding, she slipped me in anyway. In spite of that, and because I loved to study and learn the material presented to me, I became an exceptional student. I seemed to understand things before they were even taught to me. I always had the feeling that I had been down this road before. Nothing was new information. I could almost tell what was going to be on the next page in the textbook before the page was even turned. Consequently my grades were well above the requirement for a full scholarship, without which I could not have continued. Again a gift from that precious nun.

That was the beginning of a lifetime of undeserved, unsolicited, unexpected and unbelievable events and accomplishments, woven through each story, event and chapter, all leading to understandings that I could not have possibly imagined. None of which was I *qualified* to know or to do. Yet I both *knew* and *did*.

Twenty-five years ago after leaving medicine and spending three years in a theological teaching center, of sorts, I started the first alternative metabolic health care center in the United States. I knew nothing about alternative methods of heath care; I learned as I went. Before I interviewed each patient, I went into my office, closed my eyes and prayed to know what was wrong with them and what to do to fix them. From the beginning I witnessed the most miraculous healings of diseases and afflictions that could not be *touched* in traditional medicine. No one was more surprised than I at the immediate results that were happening daily. There was a sense with me at all times that if I surrendered what I *thought* I knew, asked for understand ing and waited, it would come. And it always did. No one was more "unqualified" to do what was being done.

As word got out about the healings that were happening, the pressure from the established medical community began to explode all around me. Multitudes of legal papers, hearings, and trials, accompanied by humiliations and accusations went on for several years. Still, through it all, the healings continued as I did my best to stay focused on the task set before me. While other alternative centers were being closed down and the practitioners forced to abandon their path, I found safety, security and success in adopting two essential philosophies. One was never to allow myself the luxury of a fighting spirit. He who put me on this path, who was so faithful to heal those that He sent, would certainly take care of anything that would attempt to obstruct His purpose. The second was not to take my eyes off my work. Never to look to the right or the left. Never to give power to anything or anyone except God. Never to react in fear or anger. Soon all the disruptive activity ceased and years later I found myself taking care of the very ones who, years before, had tried so adamantly to close me down!

The *metabolic* healings, the *spiritual* healings, the legal protection, all happened *in spite* of me. Finding my way on such an unusual path was also *in spite* of me. I was privileged to be there as it all happened, but only fools would believe that they were the personal progenitor of such accomplishments. I am not a Master, not a guru, not a leader. I am a student of Life 101, just as we all are.

My own non-qualifying position, coupled with the phenomenal results of the past thirty-five years, proves exactly what I hope to relate in this book. Just that each one of us is an individual, autonomous being. We are *complete* as we stand. Within we lack absolutely nothing. Within us resides all that is necessary or ever will be necessary in this life for complete fulfillment. Within us is the power to accomplish anything we desire, to heal anything that disturbs us. If we come touting all our qualifications, we will ultimately fail. But if we come realizing that we are *unqualified*, according to the expectations of our society, yet knowing our intrinsic wholeness and completeness, and trusting it, we cannot fail.

People want a hero, someone to follow, someone outside of themselves to turn to, to look up to. They flock to gurus, to spiritual masters, to successful ministries, to anyone who declares himself or herself to be above and beyond the masses. Anyone and everyone who seems to be where they are not.

But where is the man or woman who turns from all of that, who stands in quiet dignity, who has found the secrets that are locked away in the silence of their own souls? Where are they who have learned to listen, to hear, to trust, and to know that the Wisdom of God resides within them? Where are they who have found that It will indeed speak? It will indeed lead. It will direct. It will provide.

Let the pages of this book then serve as an introduction to me, my work and most of all, to all that I have witnessed and have come to understand on the path to freedom from the tyranny and enslavement of disease.

CHAPTER ONE

THE "PRINCIPLE OF LIFE"

There is a Principle established in the earth that if applied to healing—healing of the mind, healing of the body, healing of any phase of life—no matter how severe the situation may appear—would, in fact, heal.

It is this Principle, woven through the pages of this book, that I hope to communicate to those who are suffering in their lives.

This is a book discussing the "Principle of Life," if you will, that when properly understood and approached with desire and humility, will heal. It will heal bodies, minds, spirits, relationships, finances, and lives. You will find that you, yourself, have available the ability to heal whatever is disturbing your life—right now, whoever you are, wherever you are. You will discover that it was always intended for you to live in total peace, harmony—free of pain and free of disease and free of sadness. You will find that when you reach out for someone or something outside of yourself to heal you, although it may relieve the immediate problem, you will still be vulnerable to the next wave of disease, however it may manifest itself. We call this "immediate cure" vs. "long-term healing." It is the long-term healing that we are looking to address here. You will find that understanding this Principle, or tool, is simple, free and always available.

Emptying the Old To Prepare for the New

The law of physics tells us that we cannot put something into a space already filled. Jesus said that we cannot put new wine into old wineskins. Common sense tells us this is true long before we heard it in physics or in the Bible.

At the clinic we have used this understanding to successfully heal for twenty-five years now.

For instance, we cannot put nutrients into cells already full of toxic wastes. First we must remove the garbage, the toxins, then we can fill the cells with the good that they need in order to live, function and replenish. Whether these cells belong to the brain, the blood, the liver, the muscles, etc., the principle is the same.

So also, we cannot put a new thought into a mind already full of whatever it is clinging to. Especially if it is clinging to a thought that is producing the very destruction we are trying to be relieved from. First, we must be willing to set aside what we have previously believed, in order to hear clearly what is being said.

Again, we cannot correct bad behavior or turn our life into a new direction until we are willing to walk away from the present behavior. So, the truth here is that we cannot begin anew—no matter what phase of life experience—until we surrender the old. Standing empty and naked and trusting that the space that remains will be filled with that which we most desire.

This work is a result of at least thirty-five years of deep and intense searching and asking and wondering. The answer kept presenting itself to me all along the way—and while I couldn't help but notice its presence—I did not understand its message. I did not understand the Principle behind the events. Even when it was obvious, I continued to miss it. It was too simple, too available, and I was trained to look for the complicated. How could such an overwhelming problem of human suffering and horrible diseases have an answer at all? Let alone a simple one? Basically this book is meant to be educational, as well as a journey of how that information and understanding was revealed to me.

I cannot remember a time when I did not feel some type of a personal agenda against disease. I cannot remember how or when that started. Early on as a seventeen-year-old student nurse, I had pretty much known that my life would be involved in searching out some type of relief for human suffering. I believed that there was a way to eliminate it at its very root, and that I could find it, though I had no idea where to start looking. Although I never spoke these thoughts out loud, I never stopped thinking them.

Challenging the Expectancy of Disease

We, as a people, have the idea that disease is a necessary part of life which we must expect to happen at some time or another. We don't question it. In blind submission we expect it and, yet, we fear it. And we spend all our energy and effort fighting against it. We do all the things that we feel are right and proper, and hope that our efforts will be rewarded by remaining free of disease.

We pretty much live in fear of our body, as though it were an enemy, keeping us "ducking the blows" along the way. We believe that it can, with the slightest provocation, completely turn on us and devastate us. We don't realize this on a conscious level, but we actually see our body—and hold our body in thought—as though it were a tyrannical master that we must serve all our life. We work to feed and clothe and house it. We are totally subservient to the demands and necessities of this body.

We get immunizations to ward off the possibility of it getting sick. We go to a doctor and subject it to multiple tests and examinations to see if it is deciding to get sick. We spend a considerable percentage of our salaries buying insurance so we're at least financially covered when it does finally happen. Our whole existence is in some way or the other dominated by this expectation.

There is a way out of this. There are answers that will free us from being slaves to, and living in fear of, our bodies. There is a way out of spending so much time, effort, money and thought, being concerned about it.

Examining the Root Thought

Have you ever heard that, "As a man thinketh in his heart, so is he?" Or the age-old saying, "What you believe is what you will see?" We have been mesmerized into believing that disease is a part of life that can't be avoided. We have been so hypnotized into this thought that we do not question it. We are so involved and engrossed in the knowledge of diseases: their names, categorizing them, listing symptoms, areas of the body these symptoms can appear; listing organs that will fall victim . . . and all the various ways each of these different "names" can rear its ugly head and make its presence known to us. We talk about what can be done to avoid it, who is doing what and who is going where.

We are so entrenched in this whole picture, entertaining detailed outlines of such a *thought* structure. How many of us have ever stopped, put the brakes on and said, "What is this concept called disease? Where did it come from? What is this elusive enemy that comes creeping into our existence and is so incredibly destructive, to the point of snuffing out our lives, that, no matter how much effort or resistance we put up against it, or how much thought we give to preventing it, or how much insurance we take out to pay for it, still has the power to dominate our lives?"

Have we ever thought of asking where it comes from, or what it is all about? Not just individual diseases, but the entire arena? Can I live *above* or without disease as a formidable presence in my existence? Can you? Are we supposed to, or are we predestined to live in the kind of suffering that attacks or comes from our very own bodies?

Early on I began to question this. In my mind I wondered if it was all really necessary. Was there a common denominator to all disease? Though it took so many various forms and though we gave it such a variety of fancy, hard-to-pronounce names, was there a common cause? Could it be found? And if found, could we then walk away from the whole horrible picture?

Or could it be that this is a part of life that we cannot live without? And once disease seems to envelop one's existence, is there real, true relief for them? Not the kind that comes from drugs or surgeries or any of the other avenues currently employed. Those, we can agree, really have not *cured* anything at all. Is there anything that can offer permanent relief? Or do I have to "buy into" the belief that certain diseases or certain categorizations cannot be helped? Are our bodies so weak and our lives so vulnerable? Were we created to live in such a hostile environment as our own bodies?

Do I have to believe the prophets of doom who look at the x-rays and at the lab reports, or who look at the body itself, and shake their heads saying, "The statistics are . . ." or "My experience has been . . ."? Do we have to? Am I subservient to this? Can I find a way out of this? Is there something more to be known? Do I really have the whole picture?

Well, like everyone else, I started out seeing exactly what I was taught from birth, that disease is something to be fought against, an enemy. This would be the natural concept most people would carry. We spend many thousands of dollars and our whole life fighting against this concept. Millions of people make a living because of this. I did. Pharmaceutical companies are multi-billion-dollar enterprises and the greatest lobbyists in Washington.

Are there people who gain so much by the presence of disease that they would close this book before they got any further and say this is nonsense? Or would they, no matter how much they seem to gain by the presence of such a force, have the drive within them that would be willing to sacrifice *personal gain* to find a *greater solution*? Would they turn away from a possible solution by saying there is no solution . . . and say, "This is crazy"? Or are they searching for answers, too?

I believe that people who are suffering are searching. It is to those who want to explore this thought, those not afraid to come to a screeching halt and begin to question the whole thought of disease and the way it is being handled today, that I write.

So let us explore some of the things people *do* believe and have been taught, some of the things that we unquestionably embrace in our consciousness. These ideas and images that have been projected onto the screens of our minds. What is the best way to expose and explore these beliefs? By turning on the light. That is what I want to do for you, just as it has been done for me throughout this journey. I want to turn the lights on the images, forms, outlines and horrors that all humanity has accepted as reality. I want to turn the lights on some of the "golden calves," so to speak, of the religious world, as well. Things embraced without thought, or accepted as being the unequivocal truth. I want to expose how, by embracing some of these things, we doom ourselves to inevitable suffering. I want to show by exposing these well-worn doctrines and beliefs that have been passed on to us; so that we can see the obvious lack of necessity to suffer, and can see our way clear to reject it out of our experience.

I believe we are intended to live without disease, without pain, sorrow, or suffering. You say that's impossible? You say those things are necessary as a catalyst to move us on our journey, to keep our path going and to motivate us, . . . that it was preordained that we suffer so? First, I must say, that I never one time inflicted sickness on one of my daughters in order to keep them growing, maturing and developing on their path. Nor do I believe that God does this to His children, either. It was a natural, normal consequence of their existence, to gently and progressively pass from one understanding to another as they grew and developed. What I did was to prepare them the best way that I could, with

communication, education and encouragement. I also buff-
ered and protected them. I did everything that I believed was
necessary to teach and instruct in discretion and wisdom,
keeping them on a good and wholesome path. A healthy
path. But I never inflicted pain just to "keep them going."

"Keeping going" is not something we must generate.
Our path is not self-generated. We did not self-generate our
existence, therefore, we cannot self-generate our journey.
Our journey is part of this flow of Divine Energy, which we
refer to as God, or Eternal LIFE. I will use these words
interchangeably because, in my mind, they are the same.
Life in its purest form, full of glory, joy and the experience
of wonderment . . . is the Presence of God. Life, in and of
Itself. And as It flows, we are a part of It . . . like a river. We
are carried along by this river of Life into development and
into greater maturity and understanding. That is an auto-
matic propelling of Life. We do not need to have pain
inflicted upon us in order to continue in the impelling
direction It carries us.

So come with me, as I share with you the progressive
unfolding of new thoughts and understandings that were
revealed to me along my journey. Let us cease walking
through life blinded by darkness and confusion, seeing shadows on every wall and corner. These shadows become anything you imagine them to be, anything you have been
taught they are.

When my brother was very young he suffered from
asthma, horribly. He spent most of his nights under an oxygen tent, as was the customary treatment back then. There
were twin beds in his room, and the empty one was often

used as a catchall, collecting folded laundry waiting to be put away, coats and hats, etc. He would look over at those clothes and piles and see monsters, horrors and dreadful images. Before I tucked him into bed at night, I would have to clear that bed of anything that he could interpret as monsters. The last thing he would say before I left the room was, "Don't forget to close the closet door!" He saw clothes in the closet as something also to be feared. Already feeling weak and vulnerable, sick, frightened and alone, he was imagining all sorts of horrors. I would open the closet door and turn the light on every night saying, "Chris, see! There is nothing to be afraid of."

Let us together put out these fearful images we hold onto from ignorance, from a sense of insecurity, separateness and aloneness.

Let me close the closet door for you once again.

CHAPTER TWO

IN THE
BEGINNING

Wh"hen I was twenty-five years old, I found myself in an unbelievable situation. A very dark, bottomless hole, indeed. There was nowhere to go to escape, no one to go to, and no way out. This is a story, a true story, of a path of freedom, a road "less traveled," a way of escape, that appeared out of the darkest of human circumstances.

If I believed that what I saw and learned was only for that situation, and only for my own gain, I would thank God everyday, tell the story on rare occasions, and be done with it. But the path of my life has given me innumerable opportunities to apply this Principle, this discovery, if you will, and each time with the same positive results.

Conversely, whenever I would fail to utilize this understanding, for whatever reason, I would find myself once again shipwrecked upon the rocks of whatever human condition would choose to dominate my life experience.

I know and believe that this understanding is for everyone. It is a Principle of Life that will correct and restore any and all persons, in any and all situations. No matter how extreme or dreadful the picture may appear.

The Catalytic Experience

The year was 1970, and I was a registered nurse working since graduation in one of the first Pediatric Intensive Care Units in the nation. I was married to a Viet Nam Marine Corps vet with somewhat dubious emotional stability, but very nice looking; which made my emotional stability somewhat in question also.

I loved my work, adored my two-year-old daughter, and was pregnant with my second child. It is amazing how quickly one's life can change, isn't it? With a letter perhaps, or a phone call in the middle of the night. Or maybe a trip to the doctor's office. Whatever the condition, this was one of those times.

I had previously undergone surgery for the removal of my left kidney, which was deformed and diseased since birth. As the pregnancy progressed, it was thought that the remaining right kidney was taking on too much of an overload, so I was scheduled to have the birth via induction. This means that the doctors would determine when the baby would be born by giving a drug to begin labor. In the meantime, we moved to a new town about three hours away, so that my husband could start a new job—again. I resigned from my job to follow him to a place where I knew not a soul, seven months pregnant (I thought) and awaited the induction date. I arrived at the hospital early in the morning of May 25, and soon was settled in the labor room, with an IV in my arm, dripping in the chemical that would cause my baby to be born . . . whether she wanted to or not. And as it turned out, she did not.

A mistake in the calculations of my due date caused Lara to be born at seven months gestation, weighing only 2 1/2 pounds! What a disaster! What had we done?

I knew something was going wrong because what should have taken only a couple of hours was taking nearly twenty-four hours. But once started, we were forced to follow it to the end. I heard the doctor mutter something as soon as she was born like, "Oh, God, she is so puny." I waited to hear her cry, something I never heard. When I asked to see her, they whisked her by so fast that all I could see was a blur of a deep purple color, no movement, no sound. We were in deep trouble and I knew it.

This was the beginning of a life change so radical as to make the years before seem to belong to another person.

Lara was born with a lung disease associated with prematurity called hyaline membrane disease. Because the lungs had not finished developing, she was unable to take air in and keep her lungs inflated. She was taken to the Pediatric Intensive Care Unit where I had been head nurse before we moved.

During the first night she had five cardiac arrests. She was receiving 100 percent oxygen and still did not have enough oxygen to meet the demand of her kidneys and brain. Back in 1970, babies in this condition simply did not live.

I remember the senior resident came into my room the next morning to tell me that they felt it best to stop all the efforts. He asked permission to stop treatment. Even though I knew that she could not live in this condition, something inside of me would not let go. I knew that severe mental retardation was the outcome of oxygen depravation, even if she did survive the initial week. But I felt something swell up within me that I had never experienced before. Later I would call it faith, or a supernatural surge of hope. I knew down deep within my being that somehow, somewhere, someday all of this would be resolved. I had no idea what was prompting me, but I couldn't let go. I know they wished that they hadn't asked me at all. Usually they don't.

I want to stress here that I wasn't struggling to believe something. I could not have made myself feel the calm, quiet, undisturbed assurance (amidst much evidence to the contrary) that everything was going to be okay. Up until that time I knew nothing of such matters. My total reliance was on Medicine. I fully believed that this was all that was available to mankind to solve physical infirmities. I wasn't excluding anything else, such as God intervening. I just never thought about anything like that in my life. So this was an experience out of the blue.

I gave every appearance of being an emotional wreck. It was as if there were two people living inside me. One was so confident. The other, the more familiar one, was my usual hyper-frightened self, only more so. I smoked myself sick. I called the lab for results on her blood work every hour. I sneaked out of my hospital room in the middle of the night to see her, although I was warned not to do so.

What I saw that night, I would never forget. Her arms were flailing in the air as she struggled to get air into her lungs. She was still a deep purplish- blue color. As I looked at her I could feel the blood leaving my head. The room spun and I fainted.

Soon after I recovered from my initial shock, I entered the unit and put my hand into the incubator. I was overwhelmed with agony as I stroked her tiny foot. I saw the other parents who had to sit outside those windows and watch as their babies fought alone and struggled to live. Even with all the empathy I felt with the families I had dealt with in Pediatrics, never had I known pain like this. Even with that deep, underlying conviction that "everything was going to be all right" and that "don't let go" feeling, still this was unbearable pain. If I had not had that deep, strong feeling inside, I would have told them *then and there* to stop treatment, because of what I was seeing her go through and what I knew her mental status would be, even if she did live.

A few days later her father left us without a word. The responsibility accompanying such a turn of events was beyond what he wanted to deal with. We were on our own now.

As miracles go, there was a new doctor in from Germany for six months. He was here to teach the doctors in the U.S. some new techniques in the care and management of this particular neonatal problem. My daughter, Lara, was his first patient. The new type of treatment, while very difficult and time consuming, worked. The weeks became months as little by little she began to improve. However, the doctors were not at all pleased with her mental function and in a few months it was confirmed that she was severely retarded.

That was the beginning of ten hard years. Years that would completely change my existence.

By way of a little background, my family had scattered after my parents were divorced when I was twelve years old. My mother was in an institution for alcoholism, my father was who knows where. I had a sister in California busy raising her three children, and at the time I had lost all contact with my brother. I was in a town where I knew no one. So basically, I was alone with two babies, no money and no way to work. Lara was too sick, even after they let her come home, and was in need of too much constant attention for me to go back to work. I felt as though we were piecing her back together again, step by step.

No one would baby-sit her so that I could work. She looked so horrible that everyone was afraid of her. For the first year and a half she would lie in whatever position I put her in, very comfortable and relaxed, with her eyes crossed and her tongue hanging loosely out of her mouth. She never cried, she never laughed, she never responded at all. When I put food into her mouth, she would take it in and swallow it. At first, whenever I gave her formula, she would stop breathing and turn deep blue in color, since she was not able to breathe and swallow at the same time. Often when she slept she would forget to breathe and turn blue. So I slept with her on my chest all night. That way I could feel when she stopped breathing and I would jostle her a little to stimulate her breathing again . . . for a while. Those were two rough years! I've had some rough ones since then, but nothing could come near topping those!

Introduction to the "Path to Life"

It was at this point that I had an experience which started me on what I call the "Path to Life." Up until then I could hardly call what I had been experiencing, LIFE. It would be more accurately described as merely existing. This experience virtually opened up my entire spirit and being to the knowledge of God. It gave me the hope and direction that was to enable me for the rest of my life, in my personal life, in my children's lives, and in the lives of hundreds of patients I have cared for since then.

This is how it came about:

I needed someone to help me care for my babies so that I could work. We had lost our home, I had sold everything I had, and we were still without money even for food. I moved us into the basement of a nursing home. It was all I could find and they were kind enough to let us stay. It was then that I remembered a pastor and his wife, whom I had befriended several years before while caring for their daughter with cystic fibrosis. I thought that they might know someone in their church who would not be afraid to take care of Lara and Linda while I worked.

When I contacted them they seemed so happy to hear from me. They said they had heard about all that had happened to me since I last saw them, which was at their daughter's funeral. Judy, the pastor's wife, said that she had been unable to find me since I had moved. Then she said something really strange to me. She said that she believed that I had contacted her because the whole church they pastored had been praying for me. Praying that I would call so that they could help me. Now here was a switch! I couldn't get someone to help me at all until that phone call, and here was someone praying to be able to help me!

This dear lady came and picked us up that day and took us to their home. They took us to their church family and they took us into their hearts. I felt such love as I had never known before. I took in that love like someone starving would take in food. I cannot describe the aloneness, fear and abandonment that I felt up until that day. They introduced me to a new life. To a life filled with hope. They introduced me to my first Bible. They introduced me to God. Not a God separate and far away, with rules-to-live-by and impossible to please, but a real and tangible Presence, here and now, to love me and to never leave me—as I felt the rest of the world had done. I knew that day that a door had opened for me that would never shut again. Once again, here was that feeling that I had experienced the day Lara was born. Only now I could identify where it had come from. Now it had roots and a source.

They taught me how to pray, and by doing so I realized I could experience that wonderful feeling of faith and hope as often as I desired. I had found a fountain of Life, in the midst of such despair and agony.

The Earliest Experience

My first tentative footsteps on this new path happened that day while they were praying with me. This experience proved to be the beginning of many "communications and revelations," that would, unquestionably, take me from darkness into Light, on the Path that I would share with you in this book. After this day I never doubted I was being led into an understanding of something that was way beyond myself. While I haven't always understood the direction I was going, still I have never doubted that I was being led.

It was a beautiful, sunshiny, September afternoon—what we call in the North, an Indian Summer. Just as we were getting to our feet after praying, the wind began to blow. The sky became black as night, as though a storm had arrived instantly and with no warning. Everything in the house began to blow around, the curtains stood straight out from the windows. But oddly enough everyone just sat very still. It came and went in a matter of minutes. Though the experience certainly commanded our attention, no one said a word about it. They were too uncomfortable and bewildered to comment. But I knew in my heart that I had just experienced my first realization of a Divine Love that would be with me every day and forever, for I felt an undeniable *surge of Life* rush through my body, almost like a mild electrical current. I was literally enveloped by *hope*. It is this hope, which has never left me, that I wish to impart to those who find themselves as I did, in the bottom of a well of despair so deep, and with no visible way out. The lights went on in my soul that day, and, though I have occasionally allowed them to dim, they have never again gone out.

After a few months, I found a job that suited my situation better so I gathered my children and moved to a new town. I joined a new church group and for the next two years I worked the night shift in a local emergency room. A dear lady from the church stayed with my daughters while I worked. I must say that I have never in my life been as completely immersed and focused as I was during that period of time. I prayed day and night. I read and re-read my Bible. We met with this new group three times a week. Other than that, I hardly spoke with anyone. I never allowed myself the distraction. I needed to understand God—I needed my little family settled and our lives healed. My oldest daughter, Linda, though very young herself, helped me care for her little sister and we limped along.

As far as Lara was concerned, no one, including me, ever spoke of her affliction—though it remained quite obvious. I never referred to Lara as being retarded. I never said the word. Nor did anyone since the hospital days ever say it to us. No one told me not to say it. It was another very strong *feeling* I had not to *own it* for Lara. I wasn't denying it. I just wasn't concerning myself with it.

This was the fulfilling of a definite Principle toward healing, though I did not know it at the time.

CHAPTER THREE

PRINCIPLE NUMBER ONE
ON THE PATH TO LIFE
"Never 'own' your affliction."

So many times since then, and years later in my clinic practice, I would listen to people give such detailed descriptions of their problems, quoting all that the doctors had said, all the journals that they had read, going to every support group, and ever-so-proud of themselves if they had conquered the proper pronunciation of the name of the disease. Everyone they knew, knew about their problem. Somehow, the identity of who they were became wrapped up in the disease. Instead of seeing it as an intrusion into their lives, they identified with it as part of their lives. It became who they were. They gave an account of how many people were praying for them. As though God's response is based on the number of people we can gather together to pray for us. As if the "fervent prayer of *one* righteous man" would not be enough! Those folks, unfortunately, rarely recovered.

I remember one patient I took care of early on at the clinic, who refused to allow her affliction to be her identity. She came with a diagnosis of multiple sclerosis. She arrived, supported on either side by two friends, who practically dragged her in. Her "legs and arms weren't working" was all she would say. She never said the word (MS) out loud and I was warned by her friends not to either. There was this unspoken law—she would deal with it, but not *own it*. Somehow that means that while you are not about to deny it, you are not taking it into your inner conscience and allowing it to become part of you. Inside, you still feel whole and intact. You just don't let it BECOME you. She recovered rapidly. Within three months she was walking several miles each day. That was twenty years ago and she is still going strong!

There is a principle here, that to focus on the problem is to let it empower your mind and to subconsciously cling to it—never allowing yourself the possibility of release. There is a difference between dealing with what you have to deal with, and building a shrine to it.

The Fulfillment of the Principle

I never once prayed for Lara to be healed. Actually it never occurred to me to pray such a prayer, for a couple of reasons.

One was that it never occurred to me that God could

do it. As strange as that sounds for me now to say that, back then if Medicine couldn't do it—then it just wasn't going to get done. The second reason was that my whole focus was learning about God and holding my little family intact. We were in a survival mode. Most of my prayers were directed towards the next meal and the rent.

As far as Lara was concerned, the one thing that I seemed to know deep within me was that it was critical that I not give *my permission* for this thing to be part of our lives. That was about all I really knew. It may have been what we had to deal with, but it was not going to be our identity. During those first two years I was so totally immersed in my study that my spiritual consciousness really began to develop. This seemed to happen without any particular effort on my part. As a result though, many strange and wonderful things began to happen.

The most significant event was when Lara was almost two years old. The day started out pretty routine. I had no warning of what was to come. It was lunchtime and I had Lara propped up on my hip. As I started to put a piece of cracker into her mouth, she reached up and took it from me. I held my breath as she put it into her own mouth. I had not recovered from the moment when she looked right into my eyes, and she smiled at me. I will not even try to tell you the emotions that I felt. That was the first spark of recognition that she had ever shown—the first social moment of her life. There were no bells, no cymbals, and no dramatic fan-fare. Just quietly, softly and gently *awareness* slipped into her little mind and Lara was healed.

From that day on, she made rapid progress, both with

motor and social development. We still had our share of struggles for a few years, before she 'caught up' with other children her age. But eventually she did and today, twenty-seven years since that day, she is an attorney and happily married. She and her wonderful sister, Linda, are my best friends and the greatest inspiration of my life.

And that was just the beginning.

CHAPTER FOUR

THE MONKEYS
AND THE DRAGONS

Later, during that second year, I came down with pneumonia. For two weeks I dragged myself to work, then back home and collapsed. I coughed so hard that I broke two ribs on my left side, making it even more difficult to breathe. One night I stumbled out of bed and made my way into the living room. I felt that now-very-familiar *Presence* drawing me that night and I fell to my knees. I felt such a spirit of *surrender* come over me, that I lifted my hands and began to sing a song that I learned at one of our church services. Just as I started, I felt and heard a loud *snap* as the broken rib bones moved into place. The pain shot through me and I collapsed across the couch. I fell asleep and I had a dream.

In my dream I was standing on a golden path on top of a mountain, in the midst of a large mountain range, like the Alps. I saw that path winding up each mountainside and disappear over the top, only to reappear off in the distance on another mountain. I thought, "Oh, I have so far yet to go." I noticed that on both sides of the path, right at my feet, were many monkeys. They were chattering so loudly and so insistently that they were setting my nerves on edge. They were also biting at my feet and legs and making them bleed.

I was jumping and dancing around trying to shake them loose when I heard, "Don't look at them. Look straight ahead down the path." I remember how painfully difficult it was for me to look away from those scary, vexing monkeys. I was sure that if I looked away they would eat me alive! But the longer it took, the worse it became. So I finally gathered all my strength and looked away towards the path.

The instant I did, the monkeys literally became paralyzed and silent. Right in mid-air they froze. Curiosity drew me to look at them again and immediately they began to chatter and nip and bite at me—so I looked away quickly and they froze again. I did this several times, and each time with the same results. So I began to walk down the path, careful to look straight ahead. The monkeys remained *frozen* beside the path.

Suddenly, as I approached the top of the first mountain, two fire-breathing dragons appeared. They were pawing and clawing the earth as they drew closer on either side of me. They were terrifying and fierce and it was my turn to freeze. Closer and closer they came, until I was sure that they would certainly devour me. Suddenly I knew that no matter how difficult it was to make my eyes look away from them and make my feet walk on—that was exactly what I must do. With more fear than I can describe gripping at my heart, I forced my eyes away and towards the path in front of me. Immediately the dragons also froze in midair. I never looked towards them again. Staring straight ahead, with my eyes fixed on the path in front of me, I walked on to safety. When I awoke from my dream, I realized immediately that all the symptoms of disease, fever and pain were gone! I was strong and refreshed, as though I had never been sick.

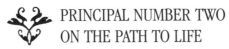 PRINCIPAL NUMBER TWO
ON THE PATH TO LIFE
*"Do not allow your situation
to mesmerize you."*

I have told this story to my patients for twenty-five years now. Everyone at the clinic knows about the "monkeys and the dragons". I hear patients telling other patients in the waiting room. I tell them, "This is a principle of LIFE. No matter how fierce the symptoms, no matter what the picture, no matter how long you have suffered— keep your eyes, your heart and your hope on the Path of LIFE before you. Though you may have to *deal with it* on some level, never become mesmerized by it. Never stare at it long enough for it to become a part of the deep-down-inside, real you."

Let me share some stories, just as they happened, that I have seen through the years in response to this principle, to enable you to better understand.

The first story is that of an elderly woman who was diagnosed with cancer of the spine and eventually sent home to die. She and her husband lived alone. He was very attentive to her, bathing her and cooking all the meals. Mostly they ate TV dinners, since he had never done the cooking before.

He knew how she loved her garden, so he moved her bed to the large bay window, and there he built for her the most beautiful flower garden. He had bird feeders and birdhouses in this garden. He even had a small fountain built with real flowing water.

They sat together day after day, week after week, watching the flowers bloom and the birds attend to their newly hatched babies. They held hands and spoke of the wonderful life they had shared together and how grateful they were for their years and experiences together. They surrounded themselves with life all around them, and let joy and gratitude fill their hearts. They did not speak of the disease. They did not speak of death.

Gradually, she began to feel stronger and soon was up cooking the meals. In time it became evident that she was healed, though, once again, they did not speak of it. Soon they were back living as before. They never returned to the doctors. They didn't feel the need to ask them if she was better, or to confirm the obvious with tests.

Their only treatment was surrounding themselves with, and enjoying the beauty of, Life. They let Life rule their hearts . . . not the predictions of death, not the images of disease. They looked at Life all day. They let the thoughts of Life fill their minds. They let gratitude fill their hearts instead of fear.

In short, though they had no idea what they were doing, they crowded death right out of their experience until all that was left was Life and wholeness. They left the monkeys and dragons behind as they stayed focused on the "Path of Life" before them.

The second story is very similar. A young couple was married just a few years when she was diagnosed with leukemia. Their religious beliefs precluded their going the conventional medical route. One of the sets of parents owned a cottage. It was out in a remote area of nature and beauty at its best. They moved there with the intention of enjoying their days together, for as long as was given to them.

Every day he carried her down to the river's edge with a blanket and a picnic lunch. They passed the days enjoying every little detail of the wonders of nature and the newness of spring life all around them. They LET Love and Life fill their hearts, living each day and being grateful for each day that came. They, also, never spoke of the problem.

Instead, they prayed and acknowledged that her life was in the hands of He, Who created her, and not at the mercy of *chance* or disease. They reasoned that they could surrender to God, but that they would *never* surrender to disease. They filled their hearts, their minds, their vision, with goodness and beauty.

She also became stronger and stronger until finally they agreed that the darkness had given way to light, and that death had given way to life. A year later they moved away from what they called "their secret place under the shadow of His wings" and continued their lives together. She remained healed.

This is also looking away from the monkeys and dragons and keeping one's eyes and vision on the Path of Life. Not in order to manipulate God to do something that we think we want, but to enjoy the Life that is ours, everyday. Regardless of the outcome. This is total surrender.

Not surrendering to the circumstances. Not surrendering to "chance," as those who hold the fatalistic view of life. Not resigning to the "inevitable." But not resisting it either. Instead, surrendering to the Spirit of Love and Life. Surrendering to the Goodness of God. Not holding in thought the popular view of God, Who is as likely to drop a bomb on us, as not. Simply surrendering to God, Who is altogether Good. Only Good.

But what exactly was this "Path of Life?" I knew that the monkeys and dragons were anything that would rob us of wholeness and happiness in any area of life. However, to begin to fully comprehend what was referred to as "the path" took many years and a multitude of experiences. I felt as though I was being taken by my hand and led from one glimmer of understanding to another—from one ray of light, to finally seeing the whole sunrise.

At this point the most frequently asked question is this, "Can one 'not surrender to the circumstances' and yet still 'deal' with the events that come crashing down on them?" In other words, "Is there ever a time when human steps must be taken while still handling the problem on a spiritual level?" And the answer is, "Absolutely." This is where Wisdom comes in, to lead and guide us through these situations. However, the impulses of Wisdom can only be heard where fear has been set aside and an internal quietness and a degree of calmness has been insisted upon.

In the preceding stories there was really nothing more to be done as far as human efforts were concerned, at least nothing that would produce a viable outcome. Unfortunately many people acquiesce to unwise, and sometimes even barbaric suggestions offered to them when faced with terrifying news. Solutions that are often worse than the original problem. They become emotionally paralyzed in their thinking—and too often those in positions of responsibility offering them their options take terrible advantage of the moment. It takes a workable relationship with Wisdom for one to see themselves through those times.

I am reminded of the young mother of a three-year-old daughter who received the news that her child had a malignant brain tumor. She was an emotionally stable young woman who was clearly accustomed to dealing with problems in a mature, well thought-out manner. After insisting on a few days to 'sort out' her thoughts, she returned to hear her options. Her reply was simple and direct. "If I agree to allow my daughter to undergo surgery, can you 'get it all' without destroying her ability to function?" When she was told that they could only remove 80 percent of the tumor and that it would return, she respectfully declined the offer. Her next question when confronted with radiation as an alternative to surgery was, "If I agree to this, will it save her life?" Sadly, they told her that it would not. Again she respectfully declined. Realizing that they were up against a thinking person who would not be swayed against reason, they didn't even offer chemotherapy. She thanked them and left with her child in her arms saying that if she needed them in the future, she was sure that they would be there for her. She took her daughter home, into the master bedroom, and closed the door behind them. She never came out or received a phone call or a visitor, nor did she discuss her situation with another soul, until the child was healed. The time involved was three months. She prayed for guidance, fully knowing that God would take them step-by-step into a viable outcome. They sang hymns, read children's Bible stories out loud, listened to the Bible read on a reel-to-reel tape while they slept at night and in general surrounded themselves with words of hope and faith and Life. Her husband did the cooking and took care of their son, as well as intercepted the visitors and calls. I was still in contact with them five years later. They never spoke of the problem and it never returned.

The issue then is not so much what one does or does not do, but *why* one is doing or not doing. Are we responding to Wisdom or are we responding to fear? Are we being led by Wisdom or by what is medically or 'religiously' expected that we should do? Are we being led by Wisdom or by what our families, friends or religious doctrines insist we must do?

By contrast, an incident happened in my own experience where my healing came through a spiritual understanding, and yet I knew that I needed medical attention to support the problem while I was learning and growing within the confines of the situation itself.

I awakened one morning after dreaming that my house was on fire. Actually, not the whole house, only the underneath part. Flames were leaping up on all sides, but strangely the house itself was not catching on fire. I ran in and out, saving as much as I could, before the floor became so hot that I could no longer run on it. As I was leaving the house for the last time, I noticed a man standing outside the front door on the porch, seemingly oblivious to the threat of smoke or flames. I stopped in my tracks and looked at him. He was so casual and nonchalant with his hands in his pockets. He spoke my name. "Michele, do not fear this event. Your house will not burn down. Your foundation will be established. Take heed of what you will see." With that I awoke and my first thought was, "Oh, now what!"

I didn't need to wait more than a second for the answer. As soon as I attempted to get out of bed, the most excruciating pain I had ever felt hit me and I fell to the floor. I was gasping for breath, my left lung felt as though it had been hit with a cannon and I was turning a dusky blue color. At the hospital it was determined that my left lung had collapsed and the pressure had shifted my heart over toward the right side of my chest. They have some fancy words for that (spontaneous pneumothorax with a mediastinal shift). Notwithstanding, that is pretty much the description of what was happening. In the emergency room they strapped me down and rammed a steel pipe-like device into my side and slid a tube into my chest, put it to an underwater seal drainage and hauled me up to the ICU, where I resided for the next two weeks. I was wired up to every conceivable machine, with tubes running in and out of me from every possible place they could find to put a tube, and some new places they made up, I think. Through it all I remembered the dream and it kept my focus away from the dreadful monkeys and terrifying dragons. Instead it kept me "centered" on the Presence and tenderness of God.

Somehow I managed to sit up, Indian style on the bed, entangled in a spiderweb of tubes and play my guitar. I sat and played and sang the same song by the hours and days. I cried a lot, but not from pain or fear. In spite of the pain, requiring numerous morphine shots, I felt an encompassing peace as I had never known before. I cried because of the extreme sense of tenderness I felt all around me. I had never before heard described such a tenderness. On one occasion I opened my eyes to find three of the nurses standing next to my bed, also crying and singing that same song with me.

I was one of the ministers at the church at the time, so I had visitors streaming in and out all day, every day. When they came I handed them my Bible and without a word spoken they would begin to read out loud to me, starting where the last visitor had left off. And so it went on day after day.

It was expected that the lung would seal itself off within three days or so. When the days became two weeks and still the situation was not resolved, I found myself facing a surgeon who announced that they were taking me to surgery the next morning to 'sandpaper' my lung. He said that the procedure would produce scar tissue that would adhere to the chest wall and artificially hold the lung up where it belonged. Inside I wondered if he had dreamed that one in a nightmare the night before. When I not-so-respectfully declined, he angrily asked just what suggestion did I have to offer? I told him that I would wait and that was all I felt that Wisdom was leading me to do.

That night I called for my good friend and fellow minister, Brother Bob, we used to call him. He and his wife arrived late, after visiting hours were over. Without a word of frivolous greeting he got right to the point. He must have been expecting my call because he knew exactly what he wanted to say. First, he asked me if I felt that God was punishing me. When I replied, "No!" He smiled and went on. Did I think that God was doing this to me to teach me something? This time I said, "Yes." He paused for a moment and softly said, "Why doesn't He just *tell* you what He wants you to know? Why hurt you to get your attention?" I realized that I had answered wrong and waited for his words. All he said to me was that I was the "Divine expression of God, Himself." That, he said, was all I needed to know.

I remember wondering if what he said was heretical and now we were really going to be in trouble! But deep inside of me, I knew the words were true. Difficult to accept, but none-the-less true. When I asked for a glass of water he answered with, "For my Lord I would do anything." When I asked for the head of the bed to be lowered he replied, "For my Lord I would do anything." The same thing happened when I asked for the oxygen to be turned down and when I asked for my morphine shot. "For my Lord I would do anything" was all he said for the remainder of the visit. When he left I fell into the deepest sleep I had experienced since my lung collapsed. I never woke until morning. I noticed two things when my eyes opened that morning. One was that the room was full of light. Not the kind of light produced by the lamps in the room, but a brilliant light. The second was a short, fat blue bird sitting on the window ledge with his head thrown back and singing for all he was worth. His song also filled the room, and filled my heart as well. It was confirmed that day that the lung had sealed. The tubes were pulled and I left for home the next day.

I would never be the same person again. I remembered the words of Jesus when He said, "If you have seen me, you have seen the Father, for I and the Father are One." I realized that day that He spoke not only of Himself but also of all the sons and daughters of God as One with Him.

CHAPTER FIVE

ROAD SIGNS
ALONG THE WAY

During the next few years I had the opportunity to be part of several healings that raised multitudes of questions in my mind. As I mentioned, I was involved in a church then. It was a group that had broken away from the standard denominations and had done some serious investigating into the Bible and the healings recorded there. I was also at this point becoming disenchanted with what was beginning to appear so barbaric to me in the treatment of diseases through the conventional medical route. The fact that regardless of the methods employed, patients were still dying of their diseases, or at best, taking drugs to enable them to live with their sufferings. I was becoming more and more interested in searching for cures, but still I knew of no other alternative, so I continued to work—now in a surgical intensive care unit.

The common medical term used when a person is healed outside of the perimeters of medical care is "spontaneous healing." Forty years ago people in medicine were loath to acknowledge God in any healings, or to give place to the spiritual element of their patients. Even so, I realized that the healings were the result of metaphysical (beyond what is seen) spiritual activity—what I now believe to be the unrestricted, unencumbered flow of something that is always present, what the Bible refers to as the Spirit of Life.

I need to relate these incidents because I feel this is what prompted me to realize that there were other avenues of healing available and to discover what they were. But, as is so often the case, instead of answering questions, these opened the door for so many more questions to be answered.

Healing the Body

One of the early healings was a young man who had fallen out of a tree during peach harvest season. This resulted in a "depressed skull fracture." Extremely depressed. As a matter of fact, the left side of his head was so caved in that his left eye was nearly lying on his cheek. Needless to say, he was unconscious. He was hooked up to every type of machine available. He had a tracheotomy tube in his throat that had developed a staph infection, so he was in "isolation." Obviously he was expected to die. Nobody was taking him to surgery or trying to change the "inevitable" outcome.

When taking care of someone in isolation, of course, one must be scrubbed, gowned, gloved and masked. The same procedure is repeated every time anyone enters the room. No one really liked working isolation because of this procedure. But it gave me a chance to be alone for awhile, so I didn't mind. I would sing the songs that I learned during the worship and praise services at church. I felt it would be peaceful for him, even though he was unconscious. I made sure the intercom to the nurse's station was turned off and I hummed and sang while I took care of him, cleaned the room, etc. Soon the room felt *alive* with a tender and Divine Love. One night after about four hours of this, I suddenly heard, "I want you to heal him."

The words were as thoughts, just bursting through my mind, interrupting whatever I was thinking at the time. There were no instructions along with those words as to how I was supposed to do this, but I got the feeling that I couldn't mess it up very badly because it was going to happen anyway!

I walked over to him and whispered what I had just heard. I put my hands on the bandages wrapped around his head and blessed him with God's healing. That was it. I went about my business and then went home.

When I returned two days later, the young man was walking in the hall supported by two people. Later they put a metal plate in his head and sent him to the VA hospital for rehabilitation. I never said anything about it to anyone at the hospital. I wouldn't have anyway because they were so against mixing medicine with religion. I understand they have lightened up on that some through the years. Nonetheless, I was amazed at what had happened and held it in my heart and wondered.

Healing the Soul

Shortly after that, we admitted a man into the unit who had been diagnosed with a Hodgkin's tumor on his spine and consequently was unable to walk. The man was angry and intimidating. He carried a holster type gun, shaved his head bald and wore a pin-stripped suit. This was Mafia country, so we concluded that he was associated with that group. Though he was reluctant at first to give up his gun, he finally did.

He yelled at everyone who walked into the room. Once he threw a full urinal at the wall in anger. He was completely bed ridden with pipe-tobacco and urine all over the sheets. Needless to say, he was difficult to take care of, and no one wanted to. The day after his surgery I went into his room and noticed that the Chaplain, or someone, had left a pamphlet on his bedside table. I picked it up and he asked me if I was "one of those religious kind of people."

I normally correct that term "religious" because it has such negative connotations with me. It brings up visions of hard-line fundamentalists, who look forward to the everlasting punishment of people not as "religious" as themselves. I certainly did not want to be associated with that kind of thought, preferring the term "spiritual," instead. But I didn't get the feeling that this was the time to make my speech on the subject, so I just said, "I believe in God."

Much to my amazement he started to cry. He asked me to tell him about God! I excused myself and went out into the hall. "God, I will do anything you ask me to do, only please don't make me talk to this man." I was just as intimidated as everyone else. But the room was *alive* with spiritual activity at that moment and I knew I was going to have to talk to him. I went back in. No matter what I prayed I was going to have to go through with this. I sat down next to him and he asked me so many questions. For an hour I answered questions with what I thought I knew, and what I had read about God.

I told him that God is Love. Not a God Who loves, but Pure Love Itself. I told him that He is not a God of punishment and pain, but that He is quick to love and heal and restore. Again, he started crying and hugging me. He asked me what he had to do to feel this Love. I told him to first be grateful that he was being led to desire this knowledge. "God's Love is evident in the fact that you want to know Him. He is the One drawing you. If you would open your heart and thank Him, you will realize that Love annihilates and washes away the past." We prayed together, using the little Bible I was given at my graduation. I gave him that Bible to read, opening it to the book of John. All day, whenever I looked in on him, he was reading that Bible. The next morning as I was making my rounds, I went in to check on him. To my astonishment I found him dead. He had evidently suffered a pulmonary embolism, common after the type of surgery that he had. He died peacefully in his sleep, still clutching that little Bible.

I stood still in that room while everyone was hustling and bustling around. I had such an eerie feeling; I could almost feel the fluttering of angel wings all around. At that moment, I had an overwhelming sense of God with me and directing me, way beyond anything I could imagine. As this was right on the heels of the first incident, I was beginning to feel that I was being carried along by some supernatural force, into who-knew-what. Again, so many questions in my mind. I felt the questions were coming faster than the answers.

Are Life and Death a Choice?

I don't believe I had an hour to get past that, when another situation came up that really rocked my understanding.

There was a woman admitted into the unit for treatment of severe rheumatoid arthritis. She was absolutely the worst case of crippling I had ever seen. She was probably in her sixties. Originally she hadn't been admitted in a dying state, though she was certainly dying now. Since all the studies performed on her were normal, no one knew why this was happening. I sat down on her bed to talk with her, to try to gain some insight into the situation, when she suddenly blurted out that she was choosing this. She said that her sisters had been caring for her and she overheard that they were taking steps to have her placed in a nursing home. She was choosing to die rather than be sent there.

I just sat there, being very young and naive. This was the first time I ever came face to face with a person who was deliberately choosing death. I was stunned. I guess up until then I had assumed that everyone would do anything in his or her power to resist death. Except in cases of frank suicide, I never knew that it could be used as an escape from other areas of suffering. At the same time I also wondered, "Could one really do that? Do we have that kind of power? Is it a choice, this living and dying? Is it our choice to make?"

What I ended up saying was, "How do you know that by choosing to run away from this challenge, you will not have to face it again somewhere along the way?"

While I thought I was being so philosophically profound, she went ballistic. This woman, who had not been able to move prior to this, sat straight up in bed. (I could almost swear I saw fangs appear and her eyes turn red). She screamed, "Get out!" She terrified me so that I flew out of the room . . . ! About two hours later she died.

This incident numbed me. I felt like I had handled it all wrong. But mostly, I had so many unanswered questions. I was convinced that there were many "behind the scenes" forces at work here, and I was somehow caught up in the midst of it all. I had no idea of much beyond that. Could people really choose death? It dawned on me that it could be true. And that by choosing, it would really happen, perhaps by disease or accident or whatever. If so, could we also in the same manner, choose to live? And that by choosing so, actually live?

Evidently, we have far more capacity to choose than I had ever realized before. I had always seen disease as victimizing people. I thought humans were helpless when disease attacked. I saw disease randomly attacking. Indiscriminately. It never crossed my mind that we might be participants in these events, and that we could somehow direct these events by choice. And if so, to what degree do we consciously, or (usually) unconsciously participate?

Of one thing I was sure; I was deliberately being led to observe these events. Also I knew that I had no personal control over these healings that took place. Another thing was, I had no idea why one person was healed in this manner and others not. This bothered me for years and it would be years later before I would understand.

Challenging the "Laws" of Disease

As I pondered these ideas of life and death, I remembered a patient I had as a student nurse. Now her story began to make more sense to me.

As a student I was somewhat of a *sponge,* soaking up every word that was taught me. I loved to learn and I was a good student. I was fascinated with medicine, every aspect of it. There was, however, an incident that happened that awakened me out of my unquestioning acceptance that everything said to me was the absolute truth.

Early on, I was taught that diseases have certain absolute characteristics and *laws* that are associated with each affliction. No matter what the disease is, there will be definite, predictable patterns and expectations accompanying that disease. It's taught that way, believed that way, expected that way, and experienced that way. It never occurred to me to challenge any of it. At that time, I would have had no reason to.

Until one day a woman was admitted to the hospital with a massive stroke. She was paralyzed on her right side and unable to talk. It was expected that she would be in that condition for the remainder of her life. The plan was to stabilize her, then send her to a nursing home for long term care until she died.

I noticed that she had no visitors, so I made a point of spending a lot of extra time with her. Soon we became great buddies. I began to notice that she would try to talk and force herself to do things that should have been *impossible* for her to do because of the stroke. I could tell that she was attempting these things in order to please me. I didn't want to encourage her because I didn't want her to be disappointed when she failed. But I never tried to stop her either. I just watched.

Early one day I was running down the hall past her room, late for "report." I waved as I flew by and then came to a screeching stop and retraced my steps. She was not in her bed, but the side rails were up and the covers still rumpled. For a second I thought that she had died during the night and I froze. Then I saw something that I never would have believed possible. She had climbed out of the bed, over the side rails and made her way across the room. She was sitting up in a chair with the proudest smile on her face. This lady progressed on to walk again and talk again, things that she should have never been able to do. She literally defied the "law" of that disease. Something motivated her, beyond the stubborn and relentless symptoms of that affliction, with all the power given it by the beliefs of man. Something like the Spirit of Life rose up within her and said, "No!"

That was a turning point in my thinking. If she could do that, what other "laws" of disease could be challenged and defeated? What factors were required? Was it available for all who would desire it? Disease with all its horror, flaunting its ugly devastation in the face of its victims, lost some of its power and substance for me that day.

CHAPTER SIX

TRANSITIONAL THOUGHTS AND EXPERIENCES

After ten years of medicine and hospital care nursing, I left for about three years and went to work as a nurse at a Theological Teaching Center/Bible School. I took care of the physical problems of the three hundred people living there and delivered all the babies. I wanted more time to be with my daughters, study my Bible, and try to find answers to my numerous questions. I realized that, for all I had heard about God, I really didn't know Him. I didn't know much more than what I heard everyone saying. I knew that the answers were going to have to come from God, Himself, and I fully expected that they would. There was a Scripture that I heard over and over in my mind in those days, "It is given unto you to know the mysteries of the kingdom of God." Believing that was true, I pressed on.

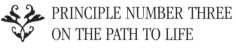 PRINCIPLE NUMBER THREE
ON THE PATH TO LIFE
"Look beyond what your eyes see."

One of the most dramatic events of that period of time was concerning a girl who was brought to the center by a relative who also lived there. Her name was Sarah. She was about twenty-five years old and had been in a mental hospital in some remote area of the country since she was three. She was put there because, for whatever reason, there was no one to raise her. I think maybe her natural mother was a patient there. Anyway, all she ever did was babble. She couldn't talk. She sort of shuffled around the grounds smiling at everyone. Everyone always greeted her with friendly hellos.

At times though, Sarah would become extremely agitated and out of control. During these times she was violent and self-destructive. She could go days and nights like this without sleeping. At one point we prayed around the clock for her, everyone taking a shift. Three hundred people with their sole focus to see this girl *whole*, and willing to sacrifice whatever it took in order for that to happen. My two-hour shift was during the middle of the night.

Just before going over to Sarah's room one night a friend of mine related a dream that she had about Sarah.

In her dream, she saw a huge oil-drum and Sarah was inside. She was so teeny-tiny inside this gigantic drum. She was banging on the side of the wall, screaming for someone to help her out of there. But the drum was so large and all the people could see was the drum. No one could see Sarah inside the drum. No one could hear her either. When I heard the dream my heart ached for her, realizing now how frightened and alone she must have felt, trapped in a body and a mind lost in hopeless insanity.

I went over to her room. She was spitting on people and cursing and babbling. She had been like that for days. I went right to the head of her bed and began to talk into her ear so she could hear me over all that noise. I realized that what we were seeing was not her real identity. The real Sarah was in there somewhere, screaming to be let out. I told her about the dream and I told her that no matter how long it took, I would stay with her until this was over. All I could see now was that frightened little girl and I knew I wouldn't abandon her. I knew that there was a perfectly normal person in there and I told her so. I told her that God heard her cries and wanted her released. "I'm not going to let go of you, Sarah. I know you hear me. I know you understand."

Everyone looked at me like I had *lost it* myself. But they also realized that something was going on and they shouldn't, and couldn't, stop me.

Sarah went wild. She broke through the straps they had across her, and went absolutely wild. It took three men falling across her to hold her down. All the while we kept singing the same song over and over.

This went on for what seemed like hours. Finally she let out the most horrible, blood-curdling scream and fell into an exhausted sleep. I remember hearing those same screams when I was training at a psychiatric hospital for six months, as a student nurse. She slept for nearly two days. When she awoke she was normal. A normal person. She stayed that way for the six months that I remained at the center.

I heard later that she was back, struggling with her original state. I don't know what ever happened to Sarah or why she seemed to relapse or how long the relapse lasted. But that incident locked in my heart forever this truth— this absolute and Divine Principle—that no matter the state a person seems to be in, no matter what they are doing or believing or experiencing on the outside—there is a whole, complete, perfect being down, deep inside. What we see on the outside is not what we need to deal with. We need to connect with the person who lives within that picture, beyond that veil. Because that person is Divine and intact. That person is whole and complete, regardless of the apparent circumstances or situations.

Now I understood the words of Jesus, in Matthew, Chapter 25, "For if you have done this to the least of my brethren, you have done it unto Me." That was a holy night and I was dealing with Someone Who was very holy.

I realized, then, how Lara was healed. There was a connection made with that whole, complete Being down within that little body. It strengthened that Being and empowered it, drawing it out into expression. The pieces of the puzzle began to come together.

CHAPTER SEVEN

PRINCIPLE NUMBER FOUR ON THE PATH TO LIFE

"Keep the river flowing."

From there I taught and ministered at a Bible School in Dallas. I was there only a short time, but I remember an incident that would add yet another piece to the whole picture.

Bonnie was also a minister at the school, who was, unfortunately, crippled and walked with a cane. Most of the time she was bedridden with pain in her back. The cause of her affliction was, at best, rather vague. But one thing was sure, Bonnie was addicted to the morphine she was taking for the pain. She had been to so many neurologists that, after a while, they refused to answer her calls. They felt that they had done all they could do for her, and they were concerned about her evident addiction.

Finally the whole Bible school decided to go into a prayer vigil for her. They did pretty much what I had seen done at the Theological Center. People were signing up for two-hour shifts around the clock. Bonnie, and another friend of mine, lived in the same apartment complex that I did.

One night, this other friend and I were praying for Bonnie together. I had shared with her some of my past experiences, and some of the things I was believing as a result. Since the understanding I had gained with Sarah was still new to me, we thought we would, once again, attempt to reach the person "down deep inside." I knew this person was still whole and complete and intact. So I sat down on Bonnie's bed and began to talk to "the Christ Being" within her. But the more I talked, just like Sarah, the more agitated she became.

I need to pause here and describe Bonnie. Regardless of the cane that she used to assist herself in walking, she seemed to *glide* wherever she went. She was so poised and *put together*. I used to wish I could be as serenely poised as she always appeared to be.

But when I began speaking to that inner person, Bonnie became hateful and bitter, quite unlike anything that she would be when she was in her *right* mind. I spoke to her and told her she was made in the image of God and that He hadn't changed His mind. That which was made in His image and likeness was, in fact, immutable. Could not be changed.

I hoped we could empower and strengthen her, and that would *throw off* this outer picture and relieve her of her suffering. We went through this most of the night and through a lot of strange activity. I just kept right on talking.

By morning though, she was healed. Not only was she pain free, but she RAN through the parking lot into the school and down the halls. She was no longer *gliding*, and so serenely poised. She was totally free and uninhibited. She was acting like anyone would act after being healed from such an enslaving existence. The whole school was wild with excitement. It was encouraging for everyone and, of course, wonderful for Bonnie.

One night about two months later, Bonnie and I were sitting together, along with about three hundred people who had come for a service at the college. The person who was supposed to give the service was ill, so they were without a preacher. The lady who ran the Bible school came up and asked if either Bonnie or I would conduct the service. Bonnie got nervous and declined so I agreed to do it.

I was speaking about discovering real Truth, as opposed to just accepting well worn, religious phrases and the "golden calves" of traditional religion. I was encouraging them not to be afraid to *not know* something—and to search out the Truth. Better to be afraid of being *duped* into believing something simply because the masses believe it. I told them to be willing to empty their hearts and come to God not knowing anything, trusting that the Spirit of Truth will teach them, "bringing them into all truth."

I was talking along these lines and the audience was as excited as I was. They were nodding their heads and clapping their hands. Everyone was with me, except Bonnie. Every time I looked at her she had her arms folded across her chest and was glaring at me. It was ugly and distracting. I found myself unable to speak when I would catch her eye, so I stopped looking at her. I recognized a tremendous jealousy. I could feel it. I had never seen it in her before, but there it was, as ugly as jealousy always is. After the service everyone was talking and hugging me, when she walked up and said, " You certainly put on quite a show." With that she turned and walked away. She never spoke with me again.

Eventually I left the college for a position in San Antonio, but not before Bonnie was back in bed, in pain, and back on the morphine.

Now what did I learn from all of that? Do I believe that God punished Bonnie for the ugliness that she allowed into her heart? Absolutely not. This is what I see.

That God is Life. And Life is like a rushing River that flows through eternity. We are in that River, whether we are in the body or not in the body. It makes no difference to the Life of the River. As we are in It, It flows through us. As long as we allow It to flow, we enjoy the many benefits and wonderful effects of the Presence of the Life. It is the energy and strength of our very existence. Sometimes, however, through ignorance or willfulness, we "choke-off" the flow of the Life. It is still flowing around us. We are still in It. But we are unable to perceive Its Presence or to feel the wonders of all Its attributes and Goodness.

When we "choke it," we feel instead, suffering. It may take the form of physical suffering, but it may, just as well, take the form of any disturbance in life. A happy heart is a happy immune system. Eyes that focus on the beauty of Life will surely see only the goodness of Life. That then will be their inheritance. But if we look through the eyes of hate, jealousy, judgement — even self-hate, or self-condemnation, we will find the ugliness and darkness that we feel in our own heart. This will make us suffer. This literally blocks the flow of Life-energy, causing a "choking down" of the flow, and a choking down of Life experiences.

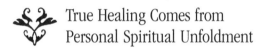 True Healing Comes from
Personal Spiritual Unfoldment

Another thing that I began to see through that incident was that in so many cases no matter who heals you, and no matter how you are healed, ultimately if it doesn't come forth from your own soul, you will have to face it again along your path until it does come from within.

As I have seen many times since these incidents, immediate relief can come through many avenues such as: being prayed for, taking medication, or being on the detoxification program which we offer at the clinic. Even running away from an impossible situation, which might be wise to do at the time.

Anyone of these, and other avenues as well, are available for us along the way. I believe they are given to us until we are better able to deal with root causes. But the day comes when our soul needs to be purified from whatever thought we have embraced, unknowingly perhaps, that might have contributed to our situation. Or when it is simply *time* for us to take the next step into a clearer understanding of Spiritual existence.

What then is to be gained by these intermediary helps? Time and maturity, a greater wisdom to handle more information and a deeper spiritual understanding.

I know in my own life, especially in my early years, one of my first reactions to situations that were intolerable to me (and there were many) was to simply remove myself. I had neither the wisdom nor maturity to handle the problems. But you can be sure that years later, as I grew in understanding and grace, I was led to *face* each situation, one by one, until I learned to *see* what God wanted me to see, and respond in Love and Strength.

Also, there were many times physical afflictions were simply taken from me through prayer. Much later though, when I would be capable of understanding better the spiritual truths that would be necessary for me to know—that understanding would allow me to eventually live *above* and without affliction, altogether.

So also, Bonnie would need to look at the negativity in her own thought, step by step ejecting each one from her soul, until she would be able to enjoy a permanent healing. This time would inevitably come for her.

This is, after all, the will of Divine Wisdom: that Eternal Love and Life be able to flow through all of creation, unobstructed and unhindered.

CHAPTER EIGHT

EMERGENCE
OUT OF MEDICINE
INTO HOLISTIC HEALING

I moved to San Antonio with the intention of helping start a Bible school, but as it turned out that was never to be. I needed to make ends meet, so I started working again in a hospital. Much time had elapsed since I last worked in the medical *school of thought*. There were so many learned experiences during those years, that the collision of different ideologies was inevitable.

The result was the beginning of my rather radical shift into "alternative" or "holistic" treatment for the relief of suffering. Though at the time I had never even heard those words spoken, and they would have had absolutely no meaning to me.

Making the transition from the medical type of thought to the holistic was really quite difficult for me. Actually I found it impossible without some serious adjustments and corrections in all that I had been taught to believe spiritually. I found that they go hand in hand and are impossible to categorize into separate compartments.

New Thought Patterns Established

In medicine we are taught always to look for and attempt to find the negative. In other words the concentration is on the disease or the abnormal. We are told to have our bodies checked at least once a year to see if everything is going well or not. We're actually afraid not to for fear something will sneak up on us and kill us, without our being aware. The intention of course is to protect us. But what it really does, is teach us that our bodies are our enemies and cannot be trusted to stay on track without our constant attention. And even then, it's a roll of the dice.

As mentioned earlier, our babies are started on a myriad of immunizations from early on. We do this because each one of us has been educated to believe that we live in a hostile world and at any given time an unseen enemy might attack. We take our babies for frequent doctor visits looking for problems because we have no confidence in the integrity of the bodies that we wear. We depend on blood studies and other related tests to tell us if we're OK.

Now please don't misunderstand. I am not attacking any of these practices. I can no longer embrace them for my own life, but I am not here to attack anything or anyone— only to show how thought patterns are established.

We learn from these, and other related practices, that the complete responsibility for the continuity of wholeness is ours. We are the masters of our own destiny. We are separate and autonomous beings, totally responsible for our lives. No wonder life, as we have thus defined it, is such a frightening experience.

No wonder we feel such tension and anxiety. This is like trying to work a multi-pieced puzzle without the picture on the box to follow. No wonder we have the high incidences of mental breakdowns, stress-related diseases, endless pill taking, and prescription drug addiction, not to mention all the other addictions we labor under.

Disease is the unseen, unknown enemy that we fear—over which we have become obsessed. We have learned to expect it, even after all our efforts to avoid it. We certainly expect it with our children using the common term, "childhood diseases" and with our elderly, "diseases of the aged" . . . diseases related to a particular type of job . . . to ethnic backgrounds . . . to certain areas of the world, etc.

We are educated to every conceivable symptom, name, and classification of disease on television, during every commercial break—always assuring us that there is a pill for every ill that is described. In short, we have been educated from birth to fear our bodies, to take extreme measures to protect ourselves, and, just in case all that doesn't work, to give voluminous portions of our earnings to insurance companies who will pay the bills (or so they say) when catastrophe strikes—as we all know that it certainly will.

If all that worldly education wasn't enough, I spent

months and years in school being taught all the names, pronunciations, classifications, appearances, signs, symptoms and descriptions of every imaginable affliction known to man—and some unimaginable ones. I learned what to look for, how to detect a problem, and what pill to give. I learned which diseases could be *masked* or controlled by which medicine; and which diseases, no matter what was done or what was cut out, would eventually win anyway.

That was the hardest *thought* of them all to *un-know* as I began in the field of holistic, alternative healing. Because in this new thought there was no such thing as "expectation of disease," let alone expectation of death by disease. Unchallenged, disease was a formidable foe. But I learned early on that the disease itself was not what was to be challenged, but the fear of it, the expectation of it, the education of it. In short, our very thought process needed to be "detoxified".

Final Days in Medicine

After moving to San Antonio in the mid 70s, I secured a position in the intensive care unit of a local hospital . . . I stayed there only one year. During this time, the internal conflict intensified between what I was doing and seeing in medicine versus what I was now knowing to be a much higher way of dealing with disease. As my understanding of spiritual truths grew, my ability to tolerate the conventional therapies waxed and waned. I began to believe that most surgeries were unnecessary, and most drugs were more deadly than the problem that they were given to correct. In the light of what I had seen over the past several years, most of the treatments seemed barbaric and unnecessary. We seemed to have lost the art of simple, common sense. Fear had so gripped the hearts of the people that they were letting anyone do anything to their bodies. I had heard of giving our bodies to medical research, but while we were still alive?

Several incidents stay in my mind as being the final "straw," so to speak. They happened within days of each other.

I will never forget little Tammy. She was six years old and had endured eighteen brain surgeries, originally for hydrocephalus (water on the brain). Most of the later surgeries were due to infection clogging up the shunt. Infection introduced at the previous surgery. She was less than her birth weight when she died. Her last days were spent lying naked on an ice mattress because of high fever, shivering and whimpering and alone. I've seen hundreds of children die in my years in pediatric ICU, but never one so brutalized.

Another memory was that of an elderly Mexican woman, who spoke not a word of English. She was admitted into the unit for severe colon bleeding. The surgeon assigned to her wanted to operate to remove her colon. But she would have no part of that. Through an interpreter, I understood her to say that she knew of a tea that would stop colon bleeding. She said that she had used it successfully for the same problem on two other occasions in her life. I related the information to the doctor who sneered and mocked her "ignorance" and insisted that I talk her and her family into the surgery. He was confident that there was no such tea. I did talk them into the operation. I will never forget the fear in her eyes. She just gave into all our demands because she felt the language barrier was too much to transcend. She was overwhelmed at the sheer force of so many pressuring her, and no one believed her anyway. After all, she was a poor Mexican woman, up against the brilliance of educated medical personnel. She never made it out of the surgery. She died on the operating table.

Later, I was to find that there certainly was, and is, a tea that is capable of stopping colon bleeding in many cases. Actually, there are several.

I couldn't help but once again question the general acceptance of what is considered *ignorance vs. educated brilliance.* I felt as though I had been manipulated into committing a crime against my own integrity.

Weeks later I was asked to scrub in for surgery on a rather difficult case. They were doing the first sex change operation in the U.S. I didn't want to be a part of that. It was a travesty against humanity in my mind and I felt I had the right to decline. The oath taken when we entered medicine was to "First, do your patient no harm." In my mind, that was harm.

Let me pause in this politically and socially correct society that we live in, to say this. I believe that people who resort to such extreme measures to relieve themselves of such intense internal conflict, do so because they see no other way out of the thought pattern that has enveloped them. I also believe that if a way of escape were presented to them, and it were true, they would take it. I do not for one minute believe, that by mutilating their bodies, they find the internal conflict resolved; but, in fact, intensified. I have counseled this situation so many times over the years to know this is true. But once again, I allowed myself to be coerced into participating in a situation that I felt was contrary to my sense of integrity.

After the operation was finished, and as I was standing over this young man in the recovery room, I could feel waves of sadness sweeping over me. I could feel the despair and isolation he lived with throughout his life and the mountain of conflict he had endured. With my heart and soul I knew, and still do, that there was a way of resolution for him that did not involve psychoanalysis or this radical and final step. In my mind this was dis-ease, as sure as any physical manifestation of dis-ease. They both have the same basic origin, the same common denominator, and the same solution. To do this to a human being, in the name of relieving suffering, was simply unacceptable.

As I stood there with these feelings filling my heart to an explosive level, another incident was brewing across the room. A very elderly woman was being wheeled into the recovery room after surgery for the removal of one of her breasts for metastatic breast cancer. Five years earlier, she had her first breast removed for the same situation. Metastases is a term used to define a cancer that has spread beyond its original borders, to some other place in the body. Now we know that as a person gets older their metabolism slows down and so does the growth of cancer. So it is generally accepted that to perform any invasive treatment on one who is well up in their years, except for an immediate life or death situation, is medically unsound. It is said that they will die of "old age" before the cancer will grow to the place of harm. Also, it is understood that once a cancer has spread to other areas of the body, there is nothing to be gained in further surgery. Another consideration was that this lady was well into her eighties and consequently would have had a serious negative effect from being given morphine for pain. So she was allowed to lie in her bed, crying and writhing in pain from the surgery.

My blood boiling over by now, I did the unthinkable and challenged the surgeon as to why he did the surgery in the first place, when he knew the obvious outcome. Before he could react to my impertinent behavior, which he certainly later did, he responded with, "Because the family expects me to do something."

With that last blow to my limping spirit, I left medicine, never to return again. I'm sure they were as glad to see me go as I was to leave.

CHAPTER NINE

A NEW BEGINNING

"Breaking the Bonds of Old Mind Sets"

A few weeks later I was introduced, by my pastor at the time, to a new urine and saliva test that was said to be able to determine the measurement of accumulated toxins in the blood and cells of the body. It was also said to show the ability of the cells to absorb nutrients. It measured the amount of accumulated toxins in the liver by determining the amount of digestive enzymes that were absent or diminished from the liver. It also showed toxic congestion of the kidneys and pancreas. The clearing of these toxins was said to allow the absorption of nutrients into the cells, and the release of metabolic wastes from the cells. This would, in turn, relieve an overburdened immune system and allow for a freer flow of Life-energy through the body.

I wish I could tell you that as soon as I heard of this I

was overwhelmed by the wonders of it. But the truth was, I pretty much thought it was somewhat nutty. I never heard of such a test. I had never heard of "toxins." So what if the system was congested? What did that have to do with disease? And what on earth was the "flow of life-energy?"

The pastor wanted me to learn the testing and how to put people on a detoxification program, believing that it would improve the health of the members of his congregation. I must admit that I was somewhat hostile to such an idea. But in time I wore down. Probably in proportion to my finances wearing down.

So, in 1976, I started the Holistic (Alternative) Health Care Clinic in San Antonio, with its humble beginnings in a local church and my "office" about the size of my bathroom at home. I learned to qualify the difference between the terms holistic and alternative treatment. Holistic simply means treating the whole person, as opposed to focusing on only one or two areas of problems within the body. In other words it is seeing the situation in conjunction with the body as a whole, interdependent unit and realizing the definite connection between the body, the mind and the emotions, as well as the spirit of the person. Alternative means treatment of a disease without the use of drugs, surgeries, radiation or any of the conventional or traditional methods now used in the practice of medicine. The term alternative could include anything from an extreme Eastern, Oriental or Indian origin to a more Western scientifically orientated approach to treatment. Because of my medical, as well as my Judeo-Christian education and background, I would probably be classified as leaning toward the more scientific approach to healing. Nevertheless, there is an immensely wide range of practice and thought encompassed in all of these terms.

Usually when people speak of Spiritual healings they are referring to recovery of health and wholeness without the aide of any human intervention at all, except perhaps through prayer, meditation and the like. I had some pretty definite distinctions in my mind of all these terms at first—but as time and experience and growth continued, the lines began to blur into a huge, single vision of Oneness, where Divine Life "enveloped it all, filled it all and was responsible for it all."

Much to my amazement, as the clinic doors opened, people actually flocked to the idea. Although we initially started the clinic for the care of the folks at that specific church, they came from miles and states and countries away.

Right from the start, I saw healings unlike anything I had ever hoped for in my wildest dreams. Who could have imagined that such horrible diseases would yield to a simple detoxification program? Lives before so crippled with affliction were responding, and so rapidly! However, even in the face of such overwhelming evidence, I still was cautious. I needed to be sure that I was doing exactly what God was leading me to do. I made a deal with God that I would never initiate a conversation about the program and I would never advertise. If this were of God, then He alone would bring the people in. He would have to be responsible. I reasoned that if I had taken the wrong turn, the people would simply not continue to come. My second deal with God was that He alone would be responsible to make the people well. (As if healing could come from another source!) As long as the diseases were "melting away" and the people were finding such relief, I would remain. But as soon as the flow started to "choke-down," or if the results became somewhat dubious, I would quit.

The reason I feel the liberty to share this information now is that after twenty-five years, I have left the clinic into capable and anointed hands, obviously raised up by God, to carry on the work. I am filled with understandings that I know, if shared, would improve the health and secure the peace of those now suffering terribly under the bondage and unlawful slavery of disease.

Before I delve too deeply into the philosophy of the work done at the clinic, and why I believe it works so well; and especially how emotions and thoughts and images that pass before our minds find their way to appearing in our bodies, I want to share with you some experiences. These finally enabled me to begin to understand what I had been looking to find all along.

Early on, the majority of my personal struggle was to try to *unknow* so much of what I had learned while in medicine. I also had to reprogram reactions and expectations to various situations and diseases. I knew that this was a whole new world and I certainly didn't need to carry into it the baggage of beliefs and fears that the patients were, themselves, trying to be rid of.

I had to learn NOT to trust in my years of experience to help me with my patients. I had to learn NOT to trust in my education and NOT to trust in the myriad of negative things that are wrong or can go wrong in any given case. I had to leave all that behind me.

I had to trust more in the "Principle of Life" as it began to reveal itself to me, and less in what my eyes saw or what my mind was outlining. There were so many opportunities for me to "see with my heart" and so many wonderful proofs of the reality of what I had chosen to believe. Before I share some of these stories, let me tell you the incident that first made me realize that in spite of all I now understood, I was still reacting to my experiences from the old mind set; the old thought pattern that kept me, as it does most of the human race, in a state of tension and turmoil. But the resolution of this experience awakened me into a new consciousness. I stepped across a chasm, never to return. I experienced a realization of the Spirit of Life, as the Life-giving Energy that flows unobstructed and unhindered through all Creation.

CHAPTER TEN

PRINCIPLE NUMBER FIVE
ON THE PATH TO LIFE

*"Realizing divine life
as the source of all life."*

I had a dear friend, pregnant for the third time, who wanted desperately to deliver this baby in her own home. This was early on when this practice was just gaining recognition. I had quite a bit of experience with home deliveries as well as my years of pediatrics, so she asked me to attend her, along with two licensed midwives. The months went by uneventfully until the day before she went into labor. It was then discovered that the baby was in a breech position (butt first). The midwives sent her for a sonogram to confirm this, and while she was in the hospital the doctor who attended her began to describe to her all the tragic things that could go wrong with this delivery at home; now that the baby was determined to be in this abnormal position. Terrified, she asked him if he would deliver the baby for her. But he told her that since he had not taken care of her up until that day, he would not assume the responsibility of delivering her child unless she submitted to a cesarean section. He expressed to her how foolish she was to have ever thought to have delivered the baby at home in the first place. Frightened and confused and angry herself, she left the hospital, still determined to have the baby as planned. That night she started labor.

They called me to come over; told me all that had happened and asked me what I thought they should do. My first response was fear, based on years of medical experience and having been thoroughly educated as to all the complications of breech childbirth. My answer was, of course, to submit to the doctor's demands and have the C-section. I felt that he was being somewhat of a jerk not to assist her in having the baby naturally—but he held the deck and he knew it. In the meantime, the midwives had arrived and were busily preparing for the delivery. They saw the conflict that the mother and the father and I were in, but they were confident that everything was in order and would go fine. Secretly I thought that they were nuts, but I couldn't deny their confidence. They seemed to know something that I didn't know, which was also a little unsettling. But the final decision was mine—all eyes were on me and I was having a world war in my head and couldn't say a word. The dad and midwives were confident. The mom wanted to do whatever I thought was best. Since it was clear that I was in a miserable conflict, and since the labor wasn't waiting for me to decide, the midwives kept getting things set up while I sat and rocked in a rocking chair and stared at the wall.

Before my mind I saw every possible problem that could arise. I remembered so many complications that I had seen in the hospital and knew that we didn't have the equipment to meet all of those problems. I knew how much the mom really wanted this home birth, and I knew that it certainly was possible that everything would go fine . . . but, what if . . . So, while I sat there in my paralyzed state of indecisiveness (a rare and uncomfortable experience for me, I might add) the baby was born. Out came one fanny cheek, which they wrapped to keep warm so the baby wouldn't feel the cold and breathe prematurely while still in the birth canal. Those girls really knew their stuff. They guided about half of the baby out, manipulated the legs out, always keeping the body wrapped with warm blankets so she wouldn't breath yet. They twisted and turned her to help the shoulders free and out came a non-breathing infant girl.

At that point I recovered from my useless state of inertia and was able to effectually resuscitate the baby. Within minutes all was quite well.

I left the room while they were finishing up, went downstairs and resumed staring at the wall. What happened? Why was I in such a state? What did they know up there that enabled them to be so calm and confident? I reasoned that they had just not seen all the horrors that I had seen in my past experience, but I wasn't sure my reasoning was right.

Soon one of them came down, sat across from me, and

began rubbing my bare feet gently to relax me. Without my needing to ask, she began to speak. "Michele, you have been trained in what we call 'human intervention.' You have been taught to expect the negative, unless you humanly jump in to fix, or divert its intention. Years of medical intervention, years of intensive care nursing, years of seeing the bad, anticipating the bad, and believing that it is the responsibility of man to redirect it—divert it—outsmart it, before 'it' strikes, has made you see yourself as some kind of a demigod, responsible for life and death. You do not trust Life. You must learn about Life. It is far more than the opposite of death. You must learn to trust it more than you trust in disease and death. You must learn to trust in Its CONTINUING PRESENCE and ABSOLUTE GOODNESS and Its ability to keep all things intact—without your help."

When I finally left later that night at about 4 a.m., I remember driving so slowly and crying all the way home. I felt that I had been awakened out of a long sleep. I felt as though I had suddenly remembered something that I had forgotten long ago. I was so grateful to finally understand, and so ashamed of my blindness and arrogance.

I knew that I had to leave all that behind me. I had to trust in Divine Life. I had to know Its unending Presence. I had to know Its utterly unchangeable nature, no matter what the human picture or human condition might be saying. I had to know its impersonal, unconditional, constant Goodness.

I had to know that Divine Goodness wasn't the least bit involved with my beliefs, or my fears, or my failures. It knows only Its own nature of pure, glorious, never beginning, never ending Life. That Life is always complete, always fulfilled, always in perfect order and harmony. And above all else, I had to know that the entire world of form and physical substance was contained within this Life. We have only to get our thoughts, our beliefs, and our fears out of the way and this unseen, but oh, so real, Life—with all Its wonders, would reveal Itself in any and every situation.

Suddenly I was faced with a choice to look away from all my previous beliefs and convictions, with all their "material-based" causes and effects and reaping and sowing principles.—and *especially* all the overwhelming personal responsibilities: to know, to fix, to fear. This now was what I had searched for. This was the explanation for all those "spontaneous healings" I had watched with such mystery and awe through so many years.

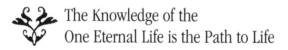 The Knowledge of the
One Eternal Life is the Path to Life

Now the body was no longer an autonomous entity deriving its life from within itself. Now I saw the body as a RESULT of the Presence and flow of Eternal Life. I note here, that this is referred to in "Eastern" healings as the Life-Energy. In our culture we refer to this Presence as God or Spirit.

If the body derived its energy and life, not from within its own being, as we have previously understood, but from the flow of this Life—Whose Presence fills all space and place—then I reasoned, I could relax all my well-meaning

efforts in avoiding catastrophe, and actually cease in my expectation of disharmony or dis-ease. It took a tremendous
amount of discipline, watching my every thought. I needed
to stay focused, always ready to correct in my thought what
was appearing (disease, suffering, chaos, confusion and disorder of every kind) with what I now realized to be the "truth
beyond the appearance." I began to look for, and actually
expected to see, Life, where there was a prognosis of death;
and to see wholeness and health, where there was only evidence of disease.

As you might expect, as I began to see Life everywhere
and in everyone, the overwhelming evidence of disease and
symptoms and misery began to disappear.

The revelation that came to me the night of the
breech delivery is the Principle of all true life. This is the
spirit and understanding that has produced the healings.
This is the Path of Life that came to me during my dream
of the monkeys and dragons. This understanding is the Path.
This now, made all things new.

CHAPTER ELEVEN

THE NEW REVELATION

The Unquestioned Proof

I will share with you two separate stories that happened as a result of this "new" revelation. These are healings that came through my deliberate insistence on the absolute nature of this Principle.

Several months later an old friend of mine, with whom I had lost touch, had suddenly fallen quite ill. Her family called and asked if I would come to the hospital and pray for her. When I arrived she was on a morphine drip and obviously in excruciating pain. Her diagnosis was acute, hemorrhagic pancreatitis. I had never heard of anyone ever surviving that condition.

That night I walked the quiet streets in the hill country where I lived. I realized I had nothing to offer my friend. My vision, my heart, was filled with medical knowledge, past experiences, morbid statistics and dark memories. Here was a situation that no one could fix. I prayed nearly all night for the grace to be able to mentally turn from it all and surrender to the truth of Life, and to my friend's permanent place in It, and It in her.

She was in surgery when I arrived the next morning. The family was gathered in the waiting room. Everyone was hugging and crying, or repeating the horrible prognosis and words of the surgeon. I knew I had to get away from that room fast if I was going to be able to hold onto the Truth of my friend, and be able to help at all.

Soon the surgeon came out and with his words and descriptions painted for me the most horrible picture. He said that all her organs had "melted down" from the pancreatic enzymes that had been released into the abdominal cavity. He said he could not tell where one organ began or another one left off. He said the whole cavity was "soup." All he did was to place several drainage tubes in her abdomen to carry off some of the dead debris. He also told us that she could not survive the devastation of this disease.

When I saw her she was all bloated up, about 100 pounds heavier than the day before, from kidney failure. She had huge dressings on her abdomen. She had tubes going everywhere and she was mercifully unconscious.

Soon I was alone with her in that room and I thought that NO MATTER WHAT THE PICTURE WAS, no matter how gruesome it appeared—in the Mind of God, whose Mind formed her in Its image and in Its likeness—nothing had really changed. Our perception of it had certainly changed. But our perception really didn't interest me anymore.

I placed my hand over those bulky dressings and as I moved my hand from one area to the other, I knew what organ or structure was supposed to be under there. I had seen perfect and intact organs hundreds of times in the past, so I chose to hold that picture in my thought, thanking God with each movement of my hand for the perfect, unchangeable form that I knew He held in His thought.

I was more "honoring God by acknowledging the truth of Life," than I was expecting to change anything. If I really believed in my heart what I knew was true in my mind, there would be nothing to change. I never spoke out loud. She never awaken during the time I was with her.

I left to join the rest of the family and within minutes a nurse came into the room where we had gathered and asked for me by name. As I stood up, she said that the patient had suddenly awakened and had asked for me to come BACK into the room! When I got there she was quite alert and smiling! She said something like, "Look what they've done to me. I'm all strapped down. The only thing I can wiggle is my behind!" And with that she began to wiggle her behind and laugh. She always was sort of a nut! As time went on she rapidly began to recover, and is today quite alive and well.

This was one of the first times I had actually witnessed what can happen when the truth is known. The truth which declares that THE SOURCE OF OUR LIFE IS NOT CONTAINED WITHIN THE BODY. IT IS NOT DEPENDENT UPON THE BODY FOR THE CONTINUATION OF ITS EXISTENCE. THE SOURCE AND ORIGIN OF OUR LIFE IS THE SAME AS FOR ALL CREATION AND IS

OUTSIDE THE PERIMETERS OF THE BODY—BUT MANIFESTED THROUGH, AND AS, THE BODY. We only need to open our hearts to the flow of this Life and to this understanding.

I had to stop looking for disease, for death around every corner. I had to look where I wanted to go. I would not drive a car looking at the houses and fields all around. I would soon be driving into those houses and fields. Instead, I would keep my eyes directly in front of me. On the road, on the path, away from the "monkeys and dragons," towards the Principle of all Life.

Continuing the Proof

Another rather dramatic proof of the continuing flow of this Divine Energy, the Spirit of Life, happened about a year later at the clinic. Each experience drove this Truth deeper into my understanding and deeper into my heart.

There was a woman who came in with a very ugly sore on the right side of her abdomen. We had a hard time communicating because she didn't speak English, but I understood from her family that she had a reoccurrence of those types of "sores" for several years. Everyone denied knowing the cause of the affliction, although they had been to doctors both in Mexico and here. They said the doctors were unable to find the cause. I found that pretty hard to understand, but they stuck to their story. I decided to put her on the "program" for two weeks and see what happened. If it had not cleared up in two weeks I would send her to a medical doctor, because I had no idea what I was dealing with. They agreed. Before the two weeks were up she was literally on her deathbed. This thing had eaten all the way around her side and deep into the abdominal wall and muscle mass. She looked like she had been holding a hand grenade when it exploded. It was a horrible sight. By then I had sent her to various hospitals in the city but they always returned, telling me that the hospitals would not take her. At first I thought it was a financial problem and I sent her to the county hospital and she still came back with the same story. I knew there was a big chunk of the story that they were not telling me, but I couldn't get to the root of it. In the meantime she was as white as a sheet with a hemoglobin of six (very low). She was gasping for air, cold and clammy. She was eminently dying.

Finally, out from under the depths of my frustration, a bolt of wisdom came. I told them to line up every medication on my desk that she was on now, or had ever been on, for this problem. They emptied her pocketbook and out came antibiotics, painkillers, sleeping medications, and anti-inflammatories. None of this was telling me anything. Then I noticed a medication that I didn't recognize called Dapson. I looked it up and found it was for the treatment of leprosy!

I shot up off my chair! Leprosy! I was so angry with them for lying to me and exposing everyone in the clinic: the staff, the other sick and weakened patients. Then, just as suddenly, all the anger went away. I remembered my new understanding. I had momentarily fallen back into the old beliefs. A calm came over me and I knew there was nothing to fear. I knew why they hadn't been telling me the truth. They had been told everywhere they went that no one could take care of her. In this country leprosy is treated in sanitariums only. Regular hospitals are not even allowed to take in leprosy patients. They believe it will expose all the other patients. That is their belief and that is the law.

I knew what they were facing and I felt sad. A warmth of love and compassion swept over me where only seconds before was a fury and anger. I told them to take their mother home and that I would pray for her. I'm sure they thought I was just dismissing them. They had no idea what I meant when I told them I was going home to pray.

That night, after I had put my two daughters to bed, I read a few Scriptures concerning leprosy. It said we were to cleanse the lepers. "Heal the sick, cleanse the lepers, raise the dead." So I thought, " Okay. This is not a suggestion. This is a command. Here I go!" Again, I had all the human thoughts about leprosy in my head, and every one of them is an obstruction to the flow of Life and healing. I knew that we all, including this dear lady, lived in the atmosphere of The Eternal Source of all Life.

My understanding is that we must first recognize this. We need to know that we derive our life-energy, our physical and mental harmony and peace from this Source. Not from within our own bodies. And that, without this, we would be inanimate objects.

Then, just as in the story of the monkeys and dragons, we must deliberately turn away from the physical evidence of disorder and disease. It's like seeing with your heart, instead of your eyes. It's choosing to see what you know is true, even though you are faced with such evidence to the contrary. Again, I needed to pray for hours to be able to see her in the light of this Truth. But every time I closed my eyes, all I could see was that horrible picture I last saw in my office. I prayed for God to see *through* me, to that which He knew was true about her. That which, in His mind, never changed. Still, all I saw was what I didn't want to see. Finally, at about 4 a.m., as my eyes were shut, I saw her on the screen of my mind getting smaller and the old picture of her shifted off to the left corner. In its place I saw a "Light Being" fill the canvas of my mind. I realized that was the true and Eternal picture of her. It only lasted a few seconds and I fell asleep.

Now let me tell you what was happening to her at the same time. Her daughter-in-law didn't want her to die in the same room where the children were sleeping so she took her back to one of the major hospitals that had previously refused to treat her. The hospital personnel knew who she was and, once again, refused to allow her back into the treatment area. So they sat in the emergency room waiting area. This unconscious woman was lying with her head in her daughter-in-law's lap and they were not going to move. The hospital staff didn't know what to do with them. Other patients came and went. Everyone just seemed to be trying to ignore them. About 3 a.m., a resident walked past them as he was leaving his shift for the night. He drove home, but by the time he pulled into his driveway he realized he just could not leave that woman lying there. He returned to the hospital. Contrary to the rules, he ordered a basement utility room to be cleared of all equipment, scrubbed and sterilized and a bed brought in for this woman. He told them to set up for sterile technique, meaning the staff had to wear gloves, masks, and scrubs which all had to be thrown away and burned when used. This is routinely done for all severe communicable diseases. They brought the woman into this room. The doctor started an IV to give her fluids and oxygen to help her breath easier. He cleaned and changed the dressing over the wound. All this was done to make her as comfortable as possible so that she could die with a little dignity and peace. He told the family he would return in twelve hours to check on her again. No one really expected her to be alive in twelve hours.

But when he returned she was conscious. In twelve more hours she was sitting up in bed and in a week she was back home. The wound healed over in two weeks—untreated, except for dressing changes. In a month she returned to Mexico. For several years, she wrote thanking me for praying that night and telling me she was doing well. At last, this new understanding was becoming dominant in my mind. I began to believe with my whole heart that this revelation could bring healing to every situation, no matter how desperate. I finally had seen too much, for too long, too consistently, to believe otherwise.

CHAPTER TWELVE

WE EXPERIENCE WHAT
WE EMBRACE IN THOUGHT

In the beginning I believed, like everyone else, that what I saw with my eyes was, of course, the truth of what was. Once this education and philosophy was embraced, life was based solely on what was seen. And that was unquestioned.

So we learn by experience and by what we're taught. We develop what we believe by what we see—what presents itself to the naked eye. A very Western thought, indeed. I was so solidly fixed in this belief that even when all the evidence to the contrary was presenting itself to me, it was years and hundreds of experiences later before I was able to understand.

More simply stated, now I understand that it is our perceptions and attitudes that determine our experiences.

What we first believe to be true, or to be reality, is what we will experience. A much more Eastern thought. First we must correct our perception and then the physical evidence will follow.

I am talking about imagination. Creating from imagery. Henry David Thoreau once stated, "Live the life you've imagined." Actually we already are! For good or ill, we are, and always have been, living out from what we are imaging. First something is seen in one's mind and then it becomes a reality.

Before one builds a building, a home, a business, even before one takes on a spouse and a family, the *dream* of it, or the imagining of it, takes place. It may be an achievement, such as climbing a mountain, excelling in a sport, or playing a musical instrument. We are told in every phase of life that to gain anything, one must first see it in one's mind. When creating, we are told to be specific. The more specific we are in our imagination concerning any particular goal, the more detailed will be our response. Even my golf instructor told me that I would never reach my goal in any given shot, unless I hold that goal in thought throughout the execution of the shot.

We are told that "we were in the Mind of God, before ever the world was framed." He also first imagined us and all creation, before it took form.

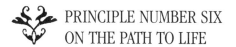 PRINCIPLE NUMBER SIX
ON THE PATH TO LIFE

"Look in the Direction You Wish to Go."

Now what do you suppose we have been doing, filling our minds and imaginations day after day with concerns of diseases, or all the efforts towards avoidance of the development of disease? From infancy on, we have been programmed towards the expectancy of disease. Or at least, towards the basic vulnerability or susceptibility to disease. With this *push* towards heredity and genetics, we're doomed before we start!

In this time of such preoccupation with the food we put into our mouths—I must say, that of far greater significance to the development of disease are the thoughts and images that are hurled at us, and that we unknowingly "eat" or embrace in our minds. So, it's not nearly so much what we eat, as what we allow to "eat us."

How can we enjoy health while all the while checking to find disease? How can we produce Life while staring at disease? Am I saying here that first we think of a disease and then we get it? No, that's pretty much nonsense. But what I am saying is that we, thinking as a collective human mind-set, carry about an UNCHALLENGED belief in our vulnerability to disease from the time we're born. We do this for ourselves and for our children. We never question the legitimacy of such expectation. We "open ourselves up" to the experience of disease, disorder, conflict and confusion in our lives and in our bodies, through allowing constant flows of negativity to pass unchecked through our thoughts daily.

There are times when we see a rash of a certain type of disease coming into the clinic after a well-known person has become afflicted with it, and the media has made a "field day" out of their situation. I remember when it was announced that a very prominent, public figure had died of lymphoma. Up until then, with all the various cancers we had seen at the clinic, we had never had a call for that particular type. I said to my partner, " Watch, now. We'll get a slew of calls with that very disease." And sure enough, we did. In just two weeks we made four appointments with that particular diagnosis.

CHAPTER THIRTEEN

THE TRUTH
THAT HEALS

At the holistic clinic we treat the body as a whole entity. We believe in the intrinsic wholeness of the organism. We focus on the order, balance and harmony of the person as a whole. From the individual cells that make up the organs and systems, to the entire structure—body, mind, soul (expression) and spiritual understanding and development. If patients can be brought into the *feeling* of wholeness, in spite of all that they have heard concerning their bodies, they can expect to regain their health.

The absolute basis of this thought is; that God, Who is Divine Intelligence and Eternal Wisdom, formed each one of us. Not as an impersonal genetic structure, as we're being told these days, but by His own imaging. We read that, "The worlds were framed by the Word of God." Each one of us was formed by His Word. Words proceed from the mind that thought them. The Mind of God thought us, imagined us, and we took the form that was imagined. He created the physical world out of what He held in His thought or Mind. So we read that we are created in His image and in His likeness. "I am the Lord and I change not," speaks of the immutable (changeless) nature of God. So, contrary to popular theological belief, we remain in that state of wonder and beauty and perfection and order. Not because we have done anything to make it so. Not because we have earned it. But solely as a result of the changeless nature of He who determined it. You only have to study the wonders of the human body to realize this is true. Except for the strange beliefs we have acquired through the many images we have been subjected to, we would enjoy the glory of such an existence. The immutable nature of God tells us that in His mind nothing has ever changed.

Because I so believe in the perfection of our being, I expect to see it manifested in each patient. I have learned through the years that the power that formed us in His image and likeness will also keep us so. I believe more in those words than in any disease that denies it.

How Thoughts Affect the Outcome of Disease

How does this all happen in our bodies? How do we let the thoughts in? How can we keep them out? What are some of the prevailing thoughts that accompany those suffering from disease? Upon what basis do we eliminate those offending thoughts?

At the clinic, many people have found health through simply keeping with the program outlined for them and their specific needs. But others, because of tenacious fears and beliefs, have inadvertently blocked their own healing, or allowed disease to reappear after it was shown to have been eliminated. Still others will experience a different disease or will have some mishap to appear later in their experience. Because of this, we spend much time uncovering the thought patterns that are often associated with sickness. What these thoughts are, and how they can be removed, always needs to be addressed with each patient.

Just as my life experience in the early years, surrounding my second daughter's birth, was a reflection of the confusion and chaos of my thought and my life, so those who come to the clinic have a foundational need for a "sense of order and balance and harmony" to be introduced first into their minds and lives, as well as their bodies. In order to establish this, many destructive beliefs and expectations must first be addressed.

Consider our body as a city set on a hill. Our mind is the wall that surrounds the city. Our spirit, the real us that lives within our consciousness, is the gatekeeper. We decide what thoughts we will allow to enter through the gates. We don't have to entertain every thought that passes by. In Bible school we had a saying, "You can't stop the birds from flying over your head, but you don't need to let them make a nest in your hair." We wouldn't allow a rapist, a thief or a murderer into our home without a fight—but we allow thoughts into our "city" that are equally destructive.

For instance, suppose we are driving down the road

and someone cuts over to our lane and nearly causes us to run off the road. The first thought that might come to us could be a response of anger at the driver's carelessness. We might even think of a derogatory name we could call him. We might in some way let him know that name. Some immediate reactions happen here. First, the fear and the anger send a message to our adrenal glands. More adrenaline is released which causes our blood vessels to constrict. This reduces the supply of oxygen to our cells allowing the cells to die prematurely, which, in turn, increases the incidence of disease. (Definite oversimplification, but nonetheless, true.) Now let's say we go to work, and we react to all the stressful incidents that accompany the day. Same story.

Now we go home and watch people killing, or in some way destroying, each other on our TV set for a couple of hours. Now a telemarketer calls. Now it's time to go to bed. All day long we have indiscriminately allowed whatever negative thoughts to enter the gates of our city. These thoughts have systematically destroyed cells, interrupted the flow of the various functions of our organs and by the end of the day our Life Energy is in the red. (The following chapter will give a detailed description of exactly how, physiologically speaking, this happens.) Now do this day after day and wonder no more why we end up with symptoms of ill health and dis-ease.

Now let's reverse the picture. As soon as the first thought of anger at that careless driver comes to our mind, we make a choice to not react with anger, but to "see through" the incident to the real person. To the unchangeable nature of the Christ, in whose image this person is created. Just because he doesn't see himself that way, and so acts in a manner impossible to the nature of God, doesn't mean that we also need to see him that way. So, we choose to act out of mercy, knowing that our safety and protection is never at the mercy of another, but always held intact by divine love and grace. And we would have rather received mercy than harsh judgment ourselves. So we bless him with a peaceful day and we calmly drive on. We choose to do this with each incident, and by the time we go home at night, we will realize such a positive flow of Life, such inner strength and such physical stamina as we have never before experienced.

The principle is that we reap exactly what we sow. What we send out, even in thought, returns to us in spades! We decide, without even realizing it, for the good that comes into our life or for the negative.

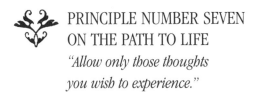 PRINCIPLE NUMBER SEVEN
ON THE PATH TO LIFE
*"Allow only those thoughts
you wish to experience."*

We have to learn to listen to the thoughts that come to us. They come to give us an opportunity for us to make a choice for life or death. People don't realize that they don't have to accept every thought that comes. Just because we hear it knocking at the door of our mind, doesn't mean that we have to "own it." We must think about each thought as it comes and decide if it is worthy to be allowed into our city. Will it bless us or harm us? It will be one or the other. We can always reject a thought and replace it with another. We are still the watchmen on the wall.

At first it may seem tedious to learn to listen to the thoughts that come. But soon with diligence and practice we will develop habits of thought and patterns of response. We will like ourselves better. We will be happier and healthier as well. We will feel more in control of our life than we have ever before realized.

The same is true about what we let in through movies, books, jokes, conversations, etc. By listening, reading or watching this, will it increase my vitality or weaken it? Absolutely everything that goes in will have some sort of an effect in our lives. This is a law of Life, a principle that we cannot escape.

In a word, what I am describing is called Wisdom. Wisdom is something that we must learn. Life cannot be randomly lived seeking only the next need to be met or the next pleasure to be obtained. Life must be well thought out and treated with respect. The beginning of Wisdom is the realization that there is a law of cause and effect, sowing and reaping. "Cast your bread upon the water and it will return after many days." This applies for the good that we would do, in thought or word or deed, or the wrong and subsequently destructive thoughts, words or deeds. Every action has a consequence. Every thought has a consequence. Much more so than we know. Disease doesn't just happen. Divorce doesn't just happen. Poverty isn't just our lot in life. While it may appear as though these things have a physical origin, I have come to realize that all true "cause" is behind the scenes—in the unseen world of thought. This will not be difficult for us to understand nor to correct in our own life.

Remember that it is the ". . . little foxes that spoil the vine." We must start with the everyday opportunities that will enable us to meet the more difficult ones down the road. Jeremiah Chapter 5, says, "If thou hast run with the footmen, and they have wearied thee, then how canst thou contend with horses? And if in the land of peace, wherein thou trusted, they wearied thee, then how wilt thou do in the swelling of Jordan?"

If we do not know what is the counter truth-thought to replace the existing negative one, we simply defer to the Mind of God. It resides within us. It is our real mind, separated from all the world thoughts that are entertained habitually. We simply silence our reactive thought, ask for the clear, pure thought or understanding of the Mind of God, and then wait for it to come. It always does.

The answers we are looking for can come only in the silence of our soul. The time to develop the habit of stopping and listening and waiting for the direction to come is now. It is far more difficult to do this when a serious crisis appears, if we have not already developed the habit. If not, we will then be swept along with the currents of the world to the same destructive results that people are currently experiencing.

CHAPTER FOURTEEN

SOME PROBLEM THOUGHTS AND BELIEFS

P eople who come to the clinic, particularly those with dreadful diseases, express thoughts of feeling as though they deserve their suffering for one reason or another. Conversely, some wonder why they are suffering when they have lived "good" lives and don't feel the punishment is deserving. This is the same belief in reverse.

Some think that life is just a roll of the dice and they have nothing to do with what has happened to them at all. We call this fatalism. Their god is "chance."

Others are so entrenched into the medical theories of heredity, contagion, etc., that they see life only as a physical cause and effect.

Let's examine the roots of some of these beliefs. This might be one of the single most important subjects we explore, because if this is not understood and cleared from thought, we will inadvertently hold onto our disease and suffering. No program on earth will be able to counter a conviction of such tenacity. Our own solid convictions will block our ability to receive the thing we pray for and desire.

Know this. All that we desire is, and has always been, available to us—always! Our receptivity is in question, not God's willingness. Divine Life is the source of our life—of all life. It is all around us and within us. We cannot get away from it if we tried. It never withholds. It does not have within Itself the nature to withhold. It is we who block our ability to receive and enjoy It. If we turn to It in our hearts, right now, and desire to understand, understanding will come.

This, right away, brings up beliefs of worthiness. Am I worthy to be sick? Am I worthy to be well? What can I do to make myself worthy? What did I do to make myself unworthy? It is enough that God or Divine Life is worthy! Believe me when I say that our own worthiness is not in question. We are not judged by our righteousness, but by His own. Most churches teach us that we must make ourselves worthy to receive anything from God. Though they vehemently deny this, still the dogma and behavioral expectations declare otherwise.

Social and employment standards hold one's worth, position and respect to be an "earned" commodity. Many parents withhold favor and affection from their children until it has been "earned." This is the social conscience that we have been born into. It has a way of keeping the recklessness and lawlessness of the human nature in harness. But God is not so. The nature and standards of God are not to be judged according to human law. Consequently, this is a rather difficult concept for people to grasp. God's judgment is according to His nature that resides deep within us, not according to our performance. The judgment of God is mercy—always. "It is the goodness of God that leads men to repentance." For those readers who are Bible scholars, re-member it is the Mercy Seat that holds a dominant posi-tion within the "Holy of Holies," covering over the Ark of the Covenant.

Nothing reaches the hardness of men's hearts with such conviction as mercy. When we know we have failed in our lives, and we feel we surely deserve punishment, and we look up to find only tenderness and mercy instead—that in and of itself, is life-changing. No one, for any reason, de-serves to be sick to "balance the score" for bad behavior.

First, on the human level we cannot change our basic human nature. We can clean it up a bit, here and there, but even then we are told that "all our righteousness is as a filthy rag." That is why we are instructed in the Bible to "reckon it dead." Reckon the old, human nature, with all its baggage, dead. This is not a "do-over." Just turn our backs on this idea of making ourselves worthy. A zebra cannot change its stripes. What we need is understanding and re-ceptivity, not worthiness.

Second, God does not see us as unworthy. He sees only what He has made. Even if we have lived our life on a level that the world deems unworthy, God sees through His own eyes, not ours. Not theirs either. We are ". . . fearfully and wonderfully made." If we are not acting like it, it's because we don't know it. We are acting out a drama, a role the way we see it. Our change will come, not when we try to make ourselves better, but when we decide to accept what God sees as true, in spite of our judgment on the subject.

The last reason that our opinion of our worthiness cannot be in question is this: Who made us to be a judge? If we are going to judge ourselves, then we are going to judge everyone else. This thought process makes us either self-condemning or self-righteous. Both attitudes are equally destructive. Remember that whatever we judge will return to us. We would do well to learn to see through the eyes of Divine Love and let that return to us. That alone will make us realize our wholeness. Remember this: ". . . for He maketh his sun to rise on the evil and on the good, and sendeth rain on the just and on the unjust." We must learn to forgive ourselves. We will be able to do that quite easily when we start forgiving others.

The one prevailing attitude at the clinic is that whatever condition or infirmity the patient comes in with is a result of the image that the world projects about life. Since the world vision is in direct contrast with the image that God holds about what He has made, we choose to believe not what we see, but what is the real, unchangeable state of Being. This gives us the confidence that we have, that with us is the Divine Love and the Eternal Wisdom of God. We are convinced that each person can and should be well. We sincerely have that expectation. For the past twenty-five years it has proven to be a solid truth to stand upon. We daily witness the most wonderful results of this, no matter the name or manifestation of the problem.

But every now and then, no matter what we know is true, no matter what type of program we devise for a patient, there still appears a resistance to the efforts. Even if one hundred times before, treating the same problem has been successful—still one or two will not respond. Or they may initially do well, only to slip back into the problem again. I realized that these people were holding certain thoughts, fears or expectations, certain mind-sets, that were blocking their own healing. In Eastern medicine, we are told that disease is any area in the body where the flow of energy is blocked. They call that congested energy. I call it "choking down" the flow of Life. It is these strange beliefs, and therefore expectations, that choke it down.

If we would stop, with all our efforts, trying to live this life the way we think we're supposed to and simply LET the Spirit of Life flow and live Its Life through us, we would find an effortless and joyful existence. A healthy one also. Remember, you who are worn out trying to please God, God is not interested in such efforts. Our very existence is a pleasure to God. He has chosen us, not the reverse.

Be still here for a moment and *feel* what it would feel like to know that God is smiling at us and loving us and pleased with us, right now. Let us forget for a minute all our judgments about ourselves, and the way we think we have failed in our life. Surely if He tells us to forgive "seventy times seventy," He does so, also. Surely if He tells us not to judge according to appearances, than neither does He.

But instead, as we are told to "see" everyone and everything that is created with eyes that "see" through the veil of mortality, to behold the wonders of Life Divine and Love unspeakable—then so does He.

And so, we must embrace the truth that "as a man thinketh, so is he." As we see ourselves as living examples of God's perfect balance, harmony and order, this perception will change our reality.

CHAPTER FIFTEEN

THE CLINIC

The clinic was the beginning effort in moving away from harsh drug therapy and debilitating surgeries. Basically the original idea was to place the body back into a condition of balance and order whereby it would heal itself. We were going back to simple basic truths about the body. We were returning to trust. Trusting the body to function in the way God intended it to at its conception in His Mind. And recognizing the presence of Divine Order and Intelligence within every cell and system.

This was the beginning of entering into the concept of non-invasive care of the body. By that we mean no longer believing that we need to automatically jump into the middle of a situation with toxic drugs or surgeries to correct a problem. But instead, gently removing whatever we recognize as an obstruction to the natural functions of the body to heal itself. Sometimes those obstructions were physical, sometimes emotional. But the greatest of all obstructions were the mental images imposed on the minds of the people. Sometimes they were the horrors of their own condition. Oftentimes, they were the horrors of the images of disease in general. Then what followed was the subsequent inability of their bodies to heal without the aid of artificial means, or, not at all.

We know that healthy thoughts and emotions have a strong and positive effect on the body. We know that negative thoughts and feelings have a definite deleterious effect on the health and strength of the body. Actually, they are an immediate drain on the strength and flow of Life-energy. But exactly how does this work? How, physiologically speaking, does this occur within the body? And how does this lead to the actual disease process? As it certainly does! By addressing this question early on at the clinic, and by discovering the answer, we have been blessed to see many and consistent healings over the past twenty-five years. Through this understanding, we have found causes of diseases that, prior to this, had no known cause. We have found how and why they have the effect in the body that they do. We have seen obvious solutions to, heretofore, impossible physical and emotional problems. We have seen lives changed and hope restored. We have seen bodies healed and homes and families healed.

What a joy for me to be involved with, what we at the clinic refer to as, " breaking the laws of disease." Every disease comes with its particular baggage of "absolutes" and "laws" connected with it. It will look like such and such.

It will act like such and such. It will progress like such and such. And then you will die right on schedule! The book of Ecclesiastes in the Old Testament of the Bible, the seventh chapter, says, "Lo, this only have I found, that God hath made man to walk upright; but they have sought out many inventions." What terrifying pictures we entertain! What a contrast with the image that God has ordained for us!

Let us now examine the physical body as it relates to health and disease, and also as it relates to its world environment. Progressively we will bridge the gap between the emotions and thoughts, and the effects of these on the physical body. We will understand exactly how "feelings" and that which we image on the screens of our minds bridge the gap over to the physical. How does something as illusive or conceptual as a thought, produce something as solid and concrete as a disease?

The Immune System

We, in medicine, recognize that the body has what we refer to as defense mechanisms—lines of defense that keep the body in a state of health. These many internal mechanisms function automatically. We don't think much about them until something goes wrong. We teach that by the time you have symptoms or have been diagnosed with a disease, these lines of defense have already broken down. We want to discover why and remove the offending cause—then build this defense system back to a state of optimum strength—thereby relieving the body of unwanted symptoms. This is commonly referred to as the immune system.

The body contains several different types of white blood cells, all working together to rid the body of accumulated toxic materials and offending microorganisms. The greater the accumulation of toxic wastes, the more white blood cells are needed to destroy and remove these offending "proteins." This process is called phagocytosis.

The immune system also includes a lymphatic system. Similar to the appearance of the blood vessels, the lymphatic system is a "river," or flowing of a thin white fluid that carries cellular waste products away from the body. If the accumulation of these wastes becomes too great, the fluid becomes thick and congested and unable to flow. You might then even find an area of swelling along the lymphatic chain. This is referred to as a congested lymph node. In order for the system to function it must be kept flushed and its purity and flow restored.

A simple way of describing this process is to once again picture your body as a castle set high on a hill. There is an army of soldiers that guards the city from within (white blood cells). There is also a wall that surrounds the city as further protection (lymphatic system). And there are centurions who stand guard as watchmen on the walls (also, a different type of white blood cell). By the time an invasion has entered the city you can readily see that several lines of defense have ceased to function as they were intended.

Prior to the advent of holistic therapy, drugs were given to treat the symptoms caused by this effect, covering over the cries of the city in an attempt to silence them, to lull them into the belief that everything was all right. The drugs, with their toxic chemicals, of course only further damaged the city. But the greatest offense was that the true problem was never addressed. Therefore, we say that they are treating symptoms and not causes. Or, as in the case of surgeries, they are cutting away the effect without dealing with the cause of the problem. So the city becomes weaker and less able to defend itself, until finally it collapses altogether. Then the disease is blamed for the final collapse, when the majority of the time the poison from the drugs, or the debilitation from extensive surgeries, was the real destroyer. Prescription drugs are listed as the fourth leading cause of death in the United States. We would list it as number one.

As medical specialization became more and more popular, the patient began to be seen as a "liver" or a "colon" or a "kidney," etc. One needed to diagnose himself first in order to know which type of special doctor to see. Your body then became compartmentalized. There was no one left who saw you as a whole being, each system interdependent with the other.

It was at this point that the drugs from one specialized doctor began to conflict with the drugs from the other specialized doctor, the right hand not knowing what the left hand was doing. Chaos and confusion resulted. The body became so drugged and toxic, it no longer was able to perform its basic function of protection and internal maintenance. Many new diseases appeared on the horizon. As a result, many new drugs also appeared.

The world was ready for a different, wiser approach;

a holistic approach (coming from the word *whole*—a single, whole unit). From the day the doors of the clinic opened, there was an overwhelming response to the holistic approach to healing and I could see that the time was right. The clinic was for the treatment of degenerative diseases. This means diseases that start from a break down within the body, as opposed to a mechanical problem, such as birth defects or trauma, meaning an accidental injury.

I entered the world of medicine in 1962, and I can tell you that easily one-half of the degenerative diseases that are commonly diagnosed today were not even known back then. With all the publicity, imaging, and descriptions out there inundating our minds with fear and expectation of disease, we have become a sick society indeed. This mass hysteria is contagious, creating after its own image.

With the advent of penicillin, most infectious diseases were finally healed or at least controlled. What a gift! I can remember people crying for joy with the news. But soon antibiotics became a panacea for every ill that afflicted man. They were freely and indiscriminately used, replacing the function of our own immune system. Rarely now can a baby get out of the newborn nursery without its first round of antibiotics. Why should the body develop its own defense system if we continually do the job for it? It is tantamount to sending in a foreign army to defend the city, instead of training the army from within its own borders. So the body then becomes dependent on antibiotics to handle its own defense. The next step is degeneration from within.

Remember how antibiotics were formed—from mold growing on a slice of bread? It was discovered that mold, when injected into the body, killed off bacteria. But what about the mold that was left behind to grow and take over? What about the healthy, *friendly* bacteria that is inadvertently killed off with the astonishing strength of the antibiotics given? This friendly bacteria is necessary for internal balance and order. Just one of the functions of the "good" bacteria is to keep down the overgrowth of disease-producing yeast found in the body. There are volumes of books and literature written about the overgrowth of this yeast, that is a direct result of taking antibiotics. Many, if not most, degenerative diseases have as their origin this overwhelming presence of "candida yeast." In Germany it was first referred to as Jerich-Hertzheimer reaction. If we research this subject, we will find that most of the new diseases that have become so prevalent today started after the advent of antibiotics. This yeast is found to release volumes of toxins within the system. Many of my patients through the years have been able to trace the beginning of their symptoms back to a time when they took a round or two of antibiotics.

Another necessity for the *friendly* bacteria is in the manufacturing and utilization of the B-Complex vitamins. These are essential for the health of our digestive and nervous systems, and are destroyed with antibiotic treatment. Do you see how with just one example of invasive treatment, so many normal bodily functions are interfered with and how many new problems are introduced into our bodies? This is just one example of how we find ourselves in the overwhelming state of chronic disease that we are in today.

The word metabolism refers to the functions of the

whole body in general, the cells specifically, and how they process their life: taking in nutrients, utilizing the nutrients, distributing that which is needful and removing the toxic wastes, and reproducing new, vibrant healthy cells. This is the primary arena of focus at the clinic. We attempt to localize where the metabolism has broken down within the cells and correct it at its cause. We have found many areas of invasion into the now, severely compromised system. Drug abuse (licensed, legal drugs) is certainly out there as a leading cause. Indiscriminate use of immunizations (too much, too young) is another; overburdening and tearing down the infant's defense system before he even has time to build it. Could this be the cause of the "illusive" sudden infant death syndrome? Many of us believe that it is.

Environmental toxins, such as lead, cadmium, mercury, copper, and aluminum are another serious and extremely prevalent source of internal toxins. Many of these are the direct cause of specific diseases. Many of these are found in our drinking water as contaminates, or metals sloughing off the walls of the pipes that transport the water. Many of these are found in the soil where our food is grown. We have found that these are not rare and isolated occurrences. But what is actually rare is to find a body that does not have at least one or more of these toxic metals present. This is another direct cause of internal breakdown.

Another common cause of internal disease is the overwhelming presence of parasites in the system. As we detoxify the body these unwanted silent guests are readily seen by the patients themselves. Most doctors in the U.S. have a tendency to deny the apparent volume of such a problem. Certainly they don't recognize this as a leading cause of many of the problems that they see on a regular basis. Part of the situation is that our method of testing for parasites here is so inferior to other countries, where the presence of parasites and their resulting diseases are more widely accepted. Isn't it odd that we are the only country that does not routinely de-worm our children on a yearly basis? Yet we do so with all our animals!

I remember on several occasions, personally carrying a jar full of parasites to labs here in this city, only to be told that it was something the patients ate! I wondered what on earth that technician ate that would make him say that! In frustration, I then would take the same jar to labs across the Mexican border to be tested for parasites. The doctors and technicians would quickly produce books with pictures of the same creatures I carried down to them. Parasites are a known, serious problem in every other country. And they are also known to be the direct cause of many symptoms and diseases, particularly digestive/intestinal and neurological. We believe that our immune system, if strong and healthy, will not allow the presence of these "foreign" substances in such prolific amounts. So the problem is once again found within the perimeters of the immune system. It is an already "compromised" system that contains a parasitical problem. We refer to these parasites as "opportunistic organisms," meaning that they gain ascendancy only after something else has worn down the immune system. So we go deeper into our discovery of cause.

I have been talking here about toxins—any unwelcome substance, regardless of the source, that resides within our bodies. There are many more that I could discuss here. But sufficient to say that toxemia, the presence of toxins in the blood—and from there into the cells—is the basic physical cause of all disease. The removal of these "foreign proteins" produces a dramatic and almost immediate response for good. Then the subsequent rebuilding effort of cell life and general overall balancing of the systems is often all it takes to see radical improvement, no matter how the disease has manifested. Anything that is degenerating can be made to regenerate. Anything.

I am going to take you on a journey inside your body, specifically your cells, as well as some of the organs in general. By doing so, I hope to educate you to the wonders of your body. I hope to introduce you to the Divine Intelligence that resides within each tiny cell and the Infinite Order that prevails throughout the entire structure. This will, I pray, help you learn something that we have all lost, something that has been swallowed up in the tidal wave of modern medicine. And that is trust. Trust in your body and trust in the Life that put it all together and holds it all together. And with that trust, comes a respect for your body, an admiration and gratitude for it, and an expectation of good.

I also want to show how the mind and the body work together. We all know that emotions cause a number of effects within the body. I want to show how all that works, the positive and the negative.

Chapter Sixteen

BRIDGING THE GAP BETWEEN THE MIND AND THE BODY

The Adrenal Glands:
Bringing the Body into Balance and Order

O_{f all the various functions of the clinic,} the basic focus is restoring the adrenal glands to functional capacity. Failure of the adrenal glands to function properly is the origin of all cellular degeneration and subsequent metabolic diseases. The adrenal glands are also the seat of all emotional responses within the body. Thus, the connection between the "drain" of negative emotions, and the advent of disease.

The adrenal glands are located above the kidneys. There are two sections to these glands, the inside area is called the medulla, and the outside layer is called the cortex. The medulla secretes one hormone only. That is epinephrine/adrenaline. This is the beginning of the stimulation of the brain and entire nervous system, and therefore, also the beginning of all the functions of the body. You know this hormone as one that responds to fear or anger, the famous "flight or fight" story. But it actually is in demand at all times, to stimulate your body into all its necessary activities. Just as adrenaline is overly triggered in the presence of hard emotions, so is it overly triggered in the presence of internal toxins, no matter what their source.

The adrenal cortex releases many hormones to produce varied functions within the body. The adrenal cortex is also subservient to the adrenal medulla. First adrenaline is secreted. That, in turn, stimulates all the hormones from the cortex. The greater the stimulation of adrenaline, for whatever reason, the more demand is placed on the cortex to produce more hormones. For the sake of understanding here, I will limit myself to discuss only two of the hormones released by the cortex, cortisol and aldosterone.

Cortisol is an anti-inflammatory hormone. It is in greater than normal demand whenever you are sick. It is in greater than normal demand if you are toxic. It is in greater than normal demand many, many times when you don't even know that you need it. It is constantly working for you, in that it is the primary stimulant to the immune system. Whenever the body needs any support at all from the immune system, it is this hormone that responds. And it knows to do so because adrenaline tells it to. This hormone also is related to the sodium electrolyte, which is critical for all the cells in the body to transport nutrients into the cells.

The other hormone from the adrenal cortex I want to mention is called aldosterone. It is responsible for the maintenance of the most critical of all substances in the cells, potassium, without which no cell would survive. Cortisol and aldosterone are married. If there is a demand for one, the other will also respond.

Normally sodium lives outside of your cells, transporting nutrients to the cell wall. Normally potassium lives inside your cells, drawing the nutrients across the cell wall into the cells. The main nutrient transported is glucose. Glucose is the food the cells need in order to live. Along with glucose, all the minerals, vitamins, etc., that the cell needs to survive are transported by way of these electrolytes, sodium and potassium.

Adrenaline stimulates cortisol and aldosterone, which motivate sodium and potassium to absorb nutrients into the cells. All of the degenerative diseases have this in common, an inability of the cells to adequately absorb and utilize nutrients (glucose, calcium, magnesium, etc.). Some of this is caused by the overwhelming presence of toxins within the cells, not allowing the absorption of nutrients. Some of this is because the sodium/potassium electrolytes are unable to do their job of transporting nutrients across the cell membrane. We call this a malabsorption at the cellular level. All degenerative diseases have both increased toxins within the cells and an interruption of the sodium/potassium balance. This causes cellular degeneration and destruction. And this is what produces the symptoms of disease.

Now what causes the imbalance of the sodium/ potassium in the cells? Remember that sodium lives outside the cells and potassium lives within the cells. Whenever adrenaline is over stimulated for whatever reason, the sodium and potassium shift positions. The potassium is shifted out of the cells into the blood stream. The sodium is shifted into the cells. This is referred to as the "sodium/potassium inversion." Nothing can enter the cells so long as sodium is "locked in." Nothing.

All degenerative diseases have this sodium/potassium inversion at the cellular level. Some much more serious than others, but always present. Now what are some reasons that this happens, and why does it happen?

Actually this is a normal process to allow us to meet the demands of whatever situation may present itself. For instance, if you are driving a car and suddenly another driver nearly hits you, you can feel the surge of adrenaline as you are maneuvering yourself out of the apparent danger. The adrenaline stimulates the adrenal cortex to produce more cortisol and aldosterone. This causes an immediate sodium/potassium shift, or inversion, at the cellular level. Since you are now in a sodium "lock in," no nutrients can enter the cells, including glucose. So glucose is diverted off the cell wall and back into the blood, causing a higher than normal blood glucose level. This increase in blood sugar allows you to be suddenly stronger than you would be otherwise. It allows you to think more clearly, and react more quickly to meet whatever demand the situation may be.

I have just described the "flight or fight" mechanism. This is one of the millions of wonderful, and constantly available, physiological processes that goes on in our bodies to maintain balance and order. As soon as the "crisis" is over, the adrenaline settles down, the cortisol and aldosterone hormones settle into their normal output, the sodium shifts back out of the cells, and the potassium shifts in.

Everything then is back to normal. All absorption is resumed and the cells begin to receive glucose and all other nutrients. What a wonderful Divine Intelligence is revealed here!

This process happens several hundred times a day and we are totally unaware of it, because of the subtle level on which it usually happens. We are only aware of it if it is of a greater than normal event or crisis. Every time we take a test this happens. If we believe that the test determines our future career, then it happens to a greater than average degree. Every time we see something on TV that triggers any hard emotion at all, we invert our sodium and potassium level and drive the blood glucose up, allowing us to deal with whatever we think we need to. And as soon as the thought or emotion is past, everything settles back to its balance and order. Or does it?

If the reason that the adrenals are overstimulated is the presence of high toxins in the body, the process of "inversion and sodium lock-in" continues relentlessly. Because of the interruption of the absorption of the nutrients into the cells, soon a person is experiencing cellular degeneration to some degree or another. When the cells are dying at a faster than normal rate, we call this "protein catabolism." All degenerative diseases demonstrate this protein (your cells) catabolism (breakdown). This is what produces the symptoms you are experiencing. Depending on where in the body the process is most felt, a specific name is given to the symptoms, and now the patient is said to have a disease.

Toxins congest the cells and block the absorption of nutrients into the cells. These toxins are a poison to the body. Again, we call this a "foreign protein" which is any substance that was not made to live in the body, no matter its origin. Parasites are a foreign protein. Prescription drugs are a foreign protein. That is why they have so many lethal side effects. Heavy metals are a foreign protein. Cells dying prematurely, as they will if the absorption of nutrients is blocked long enough, is the greatest source of foreign protein and causes the most problems.

Toxins, because they are a poison to the system, cause the adrenal glands to secrete adrenaline in a disproportionate amount, setting in motion the whole process that only further destroys the cells. The adrenal glands don't differentiate one source of stimulation from another. They respond the same if a person is angry as they would if he had, as an example, high aluminum. They don't know the difference between fear produced by a "horror" movie or watching someone you love sick and dying.

Now we have a problem, because unlike the driver who caused a temporary adrenaline rush, the toxins are present day and night. They are constantly creating the destruction of the cells and the ultimate collapse of the adrenal system from overstimulation. Watching a loved one sick, living in an unhappy relationship, working in a less than comfortable environment, all contribute to adrenal collapse. Constant worry, fear or anger will also result in an inordinate strain on the adrenal system. We call this adrenal failure or adrenal insufficiency. All degenerative diseases have this as their taproot.

So another main function at the clinic, besides identifying the toxins and removing them, is to reestablish normal adrenal function. Just removing the toxins is a great help toward that end. But dealing with the sodium lock-in and the subsequent potassium loss is another focus.

Example of Bridging the Gap

To help illustrate this, several years ago I had a patient who was a medical doctor in internal medicine. She came to the clinic with nocturnal seizures. Every morning she would wake up with blood in her mouth and all over her pillow as a result of biting on her tongue during these seizures. Incidentally, potassium is normally at the lowest level during the middle of the night, so if one is already low in the intercellular space (not necessarily in the blood) during the day, he will experience more symptoms at night.

Knowing that potassium is the main mineral for electrical conduction through the neurological system, we tested her urine, blood and did a hair analysis, to ascertain the intracellular level of potassium. Remember that when potassium shifts out of the cells it goes into the blood. So, to study only the blood to ascertain one's potassium level in the cells is not going to give an accurate picture. Blood studies are for the blood only. If you want to know what is going on in the cells, you study the urine and hair analysis. We routinely do hair analysis to find the presence of toxic metals in the cells, also. This will help us to know if that might be the underlying cause of the adrenal failure and subsequent intracellular potassium loss.

As is so often the case, this patient had a severe intracellular potassium deficit, although her blood potassium level was normal. During the course of her treatment, she checked her blood everyday to see if the dosage of potassium she was taking was causing any elevation. Much to her surprise, it never budged. But her seizures stopped immediately. In time, the underlying causes of the adrenal collapse were discovered and dealt with. In her case, the causes were some issues carried over from when her mother was dying. Also, she was unhappy with her choice of profession and finally gave herself permission to change her career to something which better suited her philosophy. She was then free of the causes of the original adrenal collapse.

Toxins are not the only physical cause of chronic adrenal failure. Infection or any inflammation will also produce an increased output of cortisol. Remember that is your anti-inflammatory hormone and the stimulus of the immune system. So any 'itis', if gone undetected or untreated, will eventually cause adrenal insufficiency. 'Itis', such as, colitis, gastritis, arthritis, hepatitis, cystitis, inflammation of the gums or tooth abscesses. Any 'itis' qualifies, no matter where its origin in the body.

To treat the person as a whole unit, both the underlying cause must be dealt with and the resultant adrenal and intercellular imbalance must be corrected. This is a basic synopsis of the work done at the Holistic Clinic. To some degree or another all alternative clinics, of any reputation at all, will deal with some of these issues. Some employ various other techniques. But the goal is to get the life energy flowing again into areas where it has been choked down, resulting in disease. And, whenever able, to determine and remove the cause of the "choke down."

CHAPTER SEVENTEEN

HOW THE
BRIDGE IS BUILT

"From the Thought to the Disease."

Now if we put all the toxins in the world on one side of a scale and we put one single hard emotion or one destructive mental image on the other side of the scale, guess which way it would tip?

There is practically not a toxin in the world more destructive to the body than one single moment of negativity. Every fear, every worry, every moment of anger or rage, every negative judgment of another or ourselves is more destructive to the body than any known toxin. And this is the reason why. When an infection or inflammation is present, the adrenals are stimulated and the entire body responds, each cell, each organ, each system doing what it was created to do to keep us in a metabolic balance. This life energy, this Spirit of Life, that flows through us, bringing Life to everything it touches and passes through, knows only

Order. It will bring order and balance to everything it comes in contact with. It causes every response of every cell to perform its function. We can count on that without our even knowing that it is happening. It will not fail to do its work successfully.

Then why are people breaking down? If the body is doing fine as a result of the Source of Life being always present, why is there disease?

When the adrenal glands are stimulated by hard emotions or any negative imagery, once the immediate "flight or fight" response is completed, there is no other activity in the body left to deal with the imbalance that is caused. We have our immune system to deal with toxins, infections, etc. We have a system in place to deal with even severe bleeding. We have a system in place to deal with choking. But except to get us out of immediate situations, there is no system in place to off-set the destruction to the adrenal glands, or the subsequent cellular destruction that takes place with every negative emotion or imagery.

We function in perfect metabolic balance when our mind and our spirit are at peace. Conflict, whatever its source, sets the adrenal glands into their overexcited mode. Unless we are able to correct that one way or another, we will suffer because of it. Thus, dis-ease.

I believe, without a doubt, that cancer derives its strength solely from the imagery that accompanies the word. It is a rare person who can be given that diagnosis who will not become paralyzed with fear from the image that is instantly drawn upon the canvas of his mind, when that word is just spoken. Then they hear how many months they have left to live. Is it any wonder that the adrenal glands experience near instant collapse? After the initial shock to the system, what then in the body is left to deal with the "foreign protein" called cancer?

Some patients, however, will not acquiesce to that scenario. They are loath to have another person tell them how and when they will die. They are loath to give disease that kind of power over them. They know that life is the flow of the Spirit of God within and through them. They know that "God only" gives life and God, not disease, will decide when they have finished what they were sent to earth to fulfill. These are the ones who come to the clinic early on, before subjecting their bodies to conventional treatments. And these are the ones who do well. Some, after first starting other treatments, decide to stop and take a more positive approach. Many of them do well also.

But those who hear the words of doom and death and believe that that is the highest sense of truth, then yield to any and every type of treatment, only to be told that they will still die from their disease—when they come as a last effort, they generally do not do well. I used to believe that they were too poisoned by the drugs to have a chance. But now I believe that they are too poisoned by the image of the disease. It is too ingrained in their minds. They come hoping, but never really expecting. This is like looking in one direction, while you are walking in another.

I want to relate a story to you that will further explain this. This is a common situation; one we see all the time. It is people, like this dear lady, who inspired the need for this book.

Helen came to the clinic with a diagnosis of severe emphysema, which she had for several years. It was becoming progressively worse, and now she was caring around an oxygen tank to help her breathe. We ran the usual tests and interviewed her extensively, as is the usual pattern for new patients. Then we devised a program for her to detoxify her body, thereby relieving the adrenal glands of the unbearable burden they were experiencing. She began her program and rapidly began to improve, as is our expectation. Within two weeks she no longer needed her oxygen to get around. She wasn't ready for a foot race yet, but I was sure that that would come later. After the initial detox, we set out to begin to reestablish healthy adrenal function, including reversing the sodium and potassium at the cellular level, so that the cells could then begin to receive nutrients and oxygen and live again. Also, reestablishing healthy adrenals will boost the immune system, thereby allowing the body to begin the process of healing itself, a function that it performs quite naturally. All the while, we continued to remove hidden and trapped toxins from the tissues and cells-especially from the liver, which stores the majority of the impurities in the body. Helen was doing great, and she continued to do great for several months.

Soon, unfortunately, her family decided to have some follow up tests done with her former medical practitioner. I suppose they wanted to *see* how well she was doing. Isn't it amazing that we have learned not to trust in what our hearts tell us is true? Unfortunately, small scattered cells of cancer were seen on x-ray within her lungs, a condition that any healthy immune system would readily be able to absorb. The fact that she looked a million times better and felt a million times better was ignored and she was told that she would die within six months. This prognosis was believed. The image hurled onto her mind produced such a paralyzing fear as to become a self-fulfilling prophecy. The adrenals shut down. The immune system shut down. Her hope shut down. The trust in the integrity of the body shut down. The flow of Life, one day before freely flowing through her body and mind and soul, choked down. All trust in the body to heal had fled. All the wonderful expectation of wholeness and health disappeared.

The very next day, after hearing this report, she came in carrying her old oxygen tank, gasping for breath, gray as a gourd, with such a look of horror upon her face. How could the disease have caused this in one day? It didn't. The imagery, the expectation, the words spoken did. How tragic that someone could look at a report and pronounce such doom and destruction and no one would challenge it. This person, this system, as it has for so many, had become their god. They feared it, they trusted it, and they completely acquiesced to it, without a word of protest. Diseases, and those declaring it, have mesmerized us all—including themselves. Helen died three weeks later.

Did the disease progress that fast? Normally, no. But with every God-given system in our body shut down from fear, perhaps. Now, do I believe that Helen's body would have been able to overcome that disease had it never been presented to her or her family? Absolutely. I have seen it too many times to doubt it. I believe that she would have continued to become stronger and healthier and, quietly and silently, Life would have been able to flow, unobstructed, to every organ and cell of the body. A healthy, happy immune system is designed to "gobble up" any and all foreign protein in the body. And cancer is a foreign protein. Only when the immune system is so severely compromised will it fail.

When I was a student nurse, I had many extra jobs to make money to be able to stay in school. One of these jobs was to assist the pathologist with autopsies. On many occasions he would point out cancers in and about the body that no one was aware of while the patient was alive. These patients had died from other causes. He was the first one to point out to me that cancer, as well as other foreign proteins, "come and go" throughout a lifetime. Our immune system is designed to deal with that and will happily do so if allowed.

My purpose for describing the work at the clinic must not be misinterpreted. I am not seeking to advertise the clinic. My goal is to enable you to clearly see how thoughts and ideas actually form physiological changes in the body, leading to sickness and disease processes. I desire to lead you to a different understanding, one that has been lost or forgotten in the flurry of excitement over human brilliance relating to medical science. It is an understanding that will break the chains of slavery to those entrapped by human suffering. If you can see how simply you fell into the "dream," then perhaps you can see how simply you can find your way into the pre-established state of absolute Divine Order.

Chapter Eighteen

IS DISEASE THE RESULT
OF MASS MESMERISM?

Through the years in my practice of holistic healing I have watched the strangest phenomena; a distinctive, yet counterproductive pattern of thought in many of my patients that I simply could not deny. While on one hand they desperately wanted a healing, on the other hand many were clinging to the thought process that provoked disease. What do I mean by that? For lack of another descriptive term I call it "mass mesmerism to an inordinate attraction to misery." Let me explain first by everyday examples that we can all identify with.

We, as a human race, seem to be drawn to the macabre. We are attracted to horror. For example, when flipping through the channels on our TV set, we come across a gourmet chef sharing his latest recipe. However, the next channel is showing a high school massacre. Which one will we be attracted to watching? Then, if we have a choice between two channels showing the same incident, but one is far more graphic in the details of the injuries, which one will attract our attention?

The classic example of this is the overwhelming ratings of the programs on TV concerning emergency room or disaster scenarios. How about the unsolved murder shows? People tell me that those shows terrorize them, but still they make a point of not missing the next program. If when driving along the highway we come across an accident, do we look at the wreck to simply manipulate our car around it, or are we really looking for bodies? Once as a paramedic nurse, I stopped at an especially morbid accident where the body of a young man was hanging outside of the window. Before we could get the wrecker truck out there to pry him loose we dodged a total of seventeen vehicle collisions due to people fixated to such a scene of horror.

Do we find ourselves listening attentively to someone's detailed description of his or her disease, or maybe his or her surgery? Or are we the one embellishing such information? The problem is that we have no idea of the destruction that is set in motion by *innocently* allowing images of negativity in our minds. Nor do we realize what we do to others when we engage in conversations that paint pictures of disease and destruction on the canvases of their minds. Most people, we can agree, are drawn to misery. Not so much from a fear of its happening to them, but more due to a strange fascination with it all. Through it all, do we have any idea what we are inviting into our lives simply by the constant imaging of such horror? Do we realize that if we spent as much concentrated time surrounding ourselves with all the wonders and beauty that the world and Life has for us, we would bring those into our lives in the same proportion? I propose that if we could get a handle on this one principle, we would dramatically reduce the incident of disease. I believe that we would also be able to see healings in many of the diseases that are on the list of the "not-able-to-be-healed."

I have an unspoken rule of behavior in my own life that says something like this: if I don't want to see something appear within the radius of my life experience, then I don't allow the words or images to start with. So I have learned and have endeavored to teach my children and patients that they are the doorkeepers to their minds. They are the "watchman on the wall" of their own city.

It is at this point that people often say to me, "I never even heard of this disease before I got it." Or, "What about children? They don't know anything about this disease." I tell them, it is not that someone thinks, "Oh, I am afraid that I will get such and such a disease," but that it is a result of being born into a collective world belief of sickness and misery—a collective world acceptance of general vulnerability to sickness. Beliefs that we are empowered to "stand against." Again, as for my own experience, I know that my daughter being born with such physical problems was a direct result of the absolute chaos and confusion of my own thought and life at the time. As I began to realize Order and Peace in my mind and heart, the external picture began to change also.

Remember that dis-ease is any condition of disorder

and disharmony, whether referring to the body, the mind, relationships, finances, etc. If order and peace are the Divine normal, than the absence of order is dis-ease. It follows then that the reestablishment of order, which produces peace, would cause disease to disappear. Much like darkness disappears with the presence of light.

If we stand and stare at disease, gasping at its horror and intensity and power to utterly devastate, we have totally empowered it over our lives. Remember the monkeys and dragons. We have given it the only power it has. We cannot hold images of disorder, disrepair, confusion, imbalance and disharmony in our minds and produce wholeness and health. This is like trying to drive to Los Angeles following a Houston map. The images that I embrace, for good or evil, become the words that I speak and the expectations in my heart, and therefore, the experiences in my life.

Early on, while seeing so clearly the law of cause and effect concerning this idea, I began to question further. In our endeavor to relieve someone of a disease, can we actually successfully eliminate one problem, but leave the "mental roots" behind to manifest as yet another branch on the same tree?

If so, I wondered, could we correct the problem called human suffering at its root? Oddly enough, I have always known deep in my heart that this was not only possible, but that I was being led, step by step, understanding by understanding, towards this end. I believe that this is the heart of God, of Divine Love, so indescribable, so inexhaustible— and that His Infinite Intelligence and Eternal Wisdom would show the way. So I trudge on, watching and wondering, listening and thinking, waiting and knowing one day we'll be there. The Mercy of God would have it no other way.

Are We Programming Ourselves to Disaster?

In the meantime, we spend all our efforts finding a reason for disease. We call it microorganisms, heredity, environmental toxins, a break down in the immune system from sadness and stress. In Western religions, we create this belief of the necessity for suffering, to move us along in our quest for a perfection that we never really expect to reach . . . seeing ourselves as evil and needing to suffer to purge ourselves of our 'inherent fallen nature'. Have you ever thought that people who act badly, even evil, are simply acting out their image of themselves? That if they were given a description of how God actually saw them, how He actually created them, they would act out that image instead?

I saw something very moving concerning this idea in Time magazine recently while reading about the Columbine High School massacre. If you remember, the students had erected crosses, one for each student slain. They also erected two crosses in memory of the two young students who had committed the murders. There were signs and scribbling all about the crosses, but one rather large sign arrested my attention. It was stretched across the crosses of the two killers and it read, "God saw you perfect, I'm sorry that we couldn't." That pretty much says it all, doesn't it?

We have built a very complicated structure surrounding this concept of suffering, and some of us defend it as though it were our nearest, dearest friend. Some misguided folks insist on a God who hurts and punishes and uses sickness to gain an expected end. They will quote their favorite Scriptures to defend such a notion, leaving one thousand Scriptures behind that declare otherwise. It is our own thoughts, beliefs and actions that hurt and punish us. It's the law of sowing and reaping, cause and effect. God is mercy. He would be delighted if we would open our hearts and receive His mercy for us right now, in spite of whether or not we think that we have deserved it, instead of living with the sense of dread that consumes us most of the time. What is mercy anyway but a kindness shown when we would deserve retribution or punishment? Also know that God would rather we have mercy for others, than a life of sacrifice of good works. "Go and learneth what that means."

Most importantly though, is there a way out of this? If one builds a structure only to find it fraught with faults, is there the courage to go back to the blueprint and make the necessary corrections? Even if it means going clear back to the basic foundation?

There are some stories that come to my mind when I talk of successfully treating an apparent disease, but not touching the mental roots and leaving so many branches of the tree behind, only to reap destruction later.

I remember early on in the practice, caring for a man who was especially dear to me and who was diagnosed with colon cancer. He was offered the usual surgical colon removal, but he refused and came to the Holistic Clinic instead. He was a good patient, did his program and never missed an appointment. In four months his medical tests revealed that the cancer was no longer evident. I remember being so excited that I jumped over my desk to give him a hug when he told me the news. He was one of the first cancer patients I had the chance to work with on the program. I think I was more excited than he was!

To describe him, Sam was without a doubt, the most eccentric human I had ever met. He owned a barbecue stand, which did quite well, in a remote little town on the outskirts of San Antonio. Everyone around knew Sam. He was enduring and lovable, but paranoid to the extreme. He carried a gun for protection, from whom I never did figure out. Before coming into the office you could find him out in the parking lot writing down license plate numbers in a notebook. He was always looking around with a suspicious expression, watching for a potential problem. I never knew who he was trying to avoid, I don't think he actually knew either. He collected antiques, junk really. He had warehouses filled with unbelievable assortments of junk. He never attempted to sell any of it, just gather it.

He also panned for gold. He would take off from the barbecue stand for a few weeks several times during the year and travel to the Northwestern part of the U.S. and live in a tent and pan for gold. Everyone who knew him loved him. Sometimes we would take turns trying to imitate his funny mannerisms. I, like everyone who knew him, thought the whole thing was kind of cute, not really to be taken very seriously.

Then one day, Sam came into my office carrying a

beat-up violin case with black electrical tape wrapped around it to hold it together. Without a word, he took out a white sheet and moved aside all the stuff on my desk to spread out his sheet. He opened his violin case and out came a gun, which he also laid on my desk (only in Texas). Then out came the strangest assortments of containers, from old socks to empty pillboxes, each one holding gold nuggets of various sizes and shapes. Before I knew what was happening, Sam had exposed his entire gold collection, totaling a net worth of well over a million dollars. He was so grateful for his healing that he wanted to give me some of his gold. I couldn't take it, of course, although I was overwhelmed at his offer.

Many months later, as the word of some of the successes we were having began to be known, and I was enduring some pressure from the medical community, Sam came by the clinic and squeezed into my hand a small package. He muttered something about my possibly needing help with my children through the conflict, and he left before I knew what had happened. The gold he left behind in my hand that day was appraised at about seventy-five thousand dollars. Over the years, we were able to use this money as a contribution to enable those patients who otherwise would not have been able to afford the treatment. However, the very next day Sam was killed in a car accident.

What a jolt! Even more than the shock of the news, I was left with such spiritual confusion (again). You see, I believed, with my whole heart that the clinic, the wisdom, knowledge and understanding in the new approach to health care, the patients that were sent to us, and every healing, was a result of the Mercy and Love of God answering the cries of the people. Now, what was the sense of healing Sam if he was going to die anyway only weeks later in an accident? Was there a root here that I had missed? Was there a much bigger healing that needed to take place? Was that true with everyone? Was his cancer just a branch on a much larger tree? Have we been treating branches all along and ignoring the taproot?

Do we see ourselves as potential victims of a hostile and changeable world? Or have we taken a stand against such common world-thought, and chosen instead to live in the Divine Love that truly does surround us. "For in Him we live and move and have our being." One of the prerequisites of any type of affliction is that we first feel small and weak in comparison to what we see as disturbing us. We feel as though we could possibly be victimized by this particular situation. For example, take the "battered woman" syndrome. Or the kid picked on at school or in the neighborhood. Or take a military officer, singling out a particular enlisted man. All of these people have one thing in common. They all believe themselves to be a victim, kind of weak and pathetic, in need of someone to take care of them or protect them. They see the world, potentially, as a hostile place to live, which could pull the rug out from under them at any time. Once a bully perceives this weakness within the victim, that is what gives him the power that he needs to overcome him. Before anyone can bully another, he must first realize a weakness, and use that as leverage. I see disease as a bully, attacking those who fear it the most. If we live in fear of anything in our lives, we give it the power it needs to overcome us.

We have not cured the *root* by only removing the battered woman from the home. Somehow she must come to a place of realization that her real enemy is her own fearful image of herself. She must be able at some point to see herself as an autonomous, self-reliant, worthwhile person. Otherwise, she will only return to her present circumstances or find a similar situation. So it is with disease. If we feel vulnerable to sickness or disease, for whatever reason, we have unknowingly opened the door for it to manifest itself. For instance, all this talk of heredity and pre-programmed genetics . . . this is the single greatest conspiracy against a sense of health and wholeness. It is programming our minds to not only expect an affliction, but to be absolutely helpless to avoid or overcome it. And you can bet we will experience it at some time or another. That is why it is so important that we begin to see ourselves, and others, as God sees us. As we were made and as we really are. And with God ONLY as our true Parent, our true Father and Mother. We derive our "genetic" inheritance from Him alone. "It is He, Who made us and not we, ourselves. We are His flock and the sheep of His pasture." We need to flee anyone who attempts to instill into our minds any idea of bodily weakness or vulnerability or susceptibility. Our strength to live *above* disease comes from the real substance of our being, not flesh and blood, but the Spirit and Life of God, freely flowing, unencumbered.

A few months later a very similar story happened. I had the privilege of caring for a gentleman who moved from a southeastern state to this area to be close to the clinic. He was suffering with coronary artery disease, so severe that he was no longer a candidate for cardiac surgery. Indeed, he was told that all the arteries in his body were so congested as to expect continuing problems with blood clots, including strokes, heart attacks, etc. He realized that, although he was still in his prime years, his days of personal productivity were over. He, also, was an exceptional patient, never deviating from his program; and an exceptional man as well. Within eight months he was running five miles a day and horseback riding three times a week. There wasn't one of us who could keep up with him. One Saturday night, he called me at home and apologized for calling so late. He said that he needed to thank me before he went to sleep that night for giving him a "new heart and a new chance at life". He cried and I cried and we hung up. The next evening, while out with his wife, a truck struck them and he was killed.

Once again, I was left with such confusion and such an empty feeling in my heart. What was I to learn from these incidents? Do we really heal people when we remove their physical afflictions only? Is there more to healing than healing the body only? Is there a mind-set towards sickness, towards death, that needs to be addressed? An expectation of negativity, even though unknown and certainly, unwanted? Do we live feeling as though we are victims of whatever this life throws at us, continually dodging the blows as they come? Is this the best we can expect? Or should we challenge this thought process? And are we created after all to live with the joy and expectation of continual care, with all our needs met before we even realize them? Living *above* the belief of being victimized by anything at all?

Closer to home, my first daughter, Linda was beset by vague, undefined fears of all sorts while she was growing up. As a baby and small child she would develop fevers and sometimes terrific pains in her feet. Our solution to this was to climb into my bed at night, (it always happened at night) and sing the songs we learned at church. After several songs, the girls would curl up to me and I would begin to pray for them. They would fall asleep almost immediately. But before they did, Linda's fever or foot pains would be gone. This probably happened over fifty times. We always did the same thing. We always experienced the same results.

At the time, I believed that God, a Supreme Being, Who I thought existed separate from Linda's being, intervened and healed Linda. Now I see it somewhat differently. Now I believe that the fears that haunted Linda choked down the flow of the Divine Life through her, and as we sang, never giving power to those fears, the flow was reestablished. Now I realize that the Divine Life is Linda's life and is our life. Now I realize that as It flows, unobstructed, we live. When It is blocked, the experience of our life, down to the smallest cell is deprived of its life energy, and dies. We kept our vision on the Path of Life, refusing to acknowledge the monkeys or dragons.

The Result of Mass Hysteria

Now comes no doubt the most poignant of all stories that tell the tale of mass hysteria surrounding disease, and the alarming consequences to such entrenching mesmerism. This is the most painful and difficult for me to tell.

While you may think this case extreme, still I have seen the same mind set over and over again, albeit on a more subtle note—but nonetheless as destructive.

This story is about my sister, Peggy, and Ray, her husband of thirty-six years. She was my only sister and because of unfortunate circumstances in our home as children, it was left to her, as the eldest, to raise our brother and me. We sort of crippled along for several years and at seventeen years old, she married Ray, who was about five years older. Together they raised three children. He worked hard and by his fiftieth birthday was promoted to vice president of a large business in upstate California. Soon the grandbabies started to arrive. Nine in all. But their joy and more-than-deserved happiness would soon come to a brutal end.

One day while mowing the lawn, Ray experienced a dull pain in his chest. Not severe, but it alarmed him. They called their family doctor and the events that followed were a blur. He was in the hospital and prepped for surgery before the sun had gone down. It was at this point that Peggy called me, hysterical and crying. Not so much because of the surgery, but because it was happening too fast and they were not given time to decide, to plan, or to think. She was especially afraid about the blood replacement problem and wanted to wait long enough for them to "harvest" his own blood. I told her to wait. To stop the whole thing. I told her that she needed to be wary of any event that is pushed upon her in a non-emergency situation. They never took the time for a breath of air. I told her that if anyone tried to push me into a decision, without first giving me time to think or pray or know what was "Wisdom" in the matter, then my answer would automatically be "no." Always.

But Peggy was different from me in many ways. She followed rules to the point of neurosis, for one thing. She trusted everyone, all the time, no matter what. It never occurred to her, nor would she have believed it, that some time people have selfish motives for doing things. She would not question authority, even if she knew something was wrong. She just blindly followed along. We teased her about this her whole life. But this time I begged her to listen to me. I felt a premonition of something horrible. Nevertheless, she agreed to the surgery.

So Ray had his heart surgery and received seven units of blood during the immediate recovery period. One year later he still had not adequately recovered and was actually in far worse shape than he had ever been before surgery. The tests revealed that Ray had contracted the AIDS virus via the blood replacement. By this time Peg was also HIV positive.

In what I refer to as blind hysteria, she obediently took drugs, knowing that they would not cure her, or even prolong her life. They made her so sick and so anemic, as to precipitate the very symptoms that finally diagnose one as having full-blown AIDS. I pleaded with her not to take them. I read the side effects to her. I sent her articles written by people with HIV, who refused to drug their bodies. They chose, rather, to place themselves on a metabolic program to build the immune system, instead of deliberately tearing it down. Many of them were doing fine after several years. Many said that they never felt stronger in their lives. Some shared documented proof that they were no longer HIV positive.

Though her doctor could offer her no hope with his treatment, still she didn't want to try anything else. Now, when people are told that they will die and the offered treatment will not work, why continue? I have watched this my whole life, and the only answer must be fear, so great, as to produce blind hysteria. Hysteria doesn't necessarily manifest as loud, wild, aggressive behavior. Many times it literally paralyzes the person. That's how it was for Peg. She rarely spoke, responding in one-word answers. Instead of reading the information, coming and talking with those who had done well on immunological building programs, she chose "support groups." They sat around and spoke of who had died since their last meeting. They talked about how sick they were and which drugs they were taking. I tried to tell her that she was focusing on the negative. She was surrounding herself with the expectation of suffering and death. She was paralyzed . . . staring at the monkeys and dragons. I may as well have been talking to a wall.

There was one incident that I had hoped would shake her from her hypnotic state. She developed the pneumonia that is common to patients with this diagnosis. Actually, she got it off and on for about a year or more. While everyone was blaming the disease, I was blaming the drugs for depressing the immune system, which is the natural process of the body to resist infectious diseases. This was a head on collision between the traditional approach to disease and the holistic approach. Without her cooperation, I was in for the ride of my life.

One day I received a call at the clinic telling me that her lung had collapsed and that she was not expected to live much longer. On the flight out there, I was reading a book by Joel Goldsmith, called, *The Art of Spiritual Healing*. I was tremendously encouraged by the time I got to the hospital. It was about one or two in the morning when I arrived. I took one look at her and felt my blood turn to ice. The devastation visited upon her little body was more than I could bear. No human being could ever "need this" suffering for any reason. I felt as though everything in me was going to explode all over the room. There was even a moment when I was blinded and everything went black. Somehow, by the Grace of God, I gathered myself together, crawled in bed with her, and started to read that book out loud. I read for eight solid hours without stopping. I knew the enemy wasn't the stupid disease. Disease doesn't have the power to destroy whatever God has made. I used to think that disease was the enemy. For years I thought that. But that was long ago. Now I knew that the enemy was blind mesmerism and blind hysteria. World belief. All that we had been conditioned to see and expect. All the fearful images that consumed our hearts and minds.

So I read the words that contradicted it all. I read out loud the words that glorified God as our Life. Words that refused to give away power that belonged to Divine Life and Eternal Love. The nurses were great. They would come in to attend to Peg and smile at me as I read on. Some of them even came over and hugged me. I was on a mission. If I couldn't save my sister, at least I was not going to acquiesce to any disease. I was going to glorify God, as the Omnipotent Presence that He says He is. I would not look at the dragons, but stay focused on the "Path of Life."

At about nine in the morning she regained consciousness and saw that I was there. I rocked her and hugged her and rubbed that bald head. Soon she was sitting on the side of the bed, and before long she was walking to the bathroom with help. That evening, much to everyone's amazement, the doctor discharged her and we took her home. Chest tube and all.

I had so hoped that that incident would change her approach to the situation. Actually, it seemed to for about a year. She began to read her Bible a little. Still she never "let go" of the disease. She often asked me why God was punishing her. She was a devout church member all her life. She attended the church that we were born into. They embraced the concept that all suffering was "The Will of God." They even told her that she was privileged to suffer for God. I attributed her confusion, and inability to embrace hope, to a life-long immersion into such thought. Nothing I said reached her. Nothing I read to her got past her confusion.

Ray, on the other hand was excited about the information. He spoke to several people in the U.S. who had followed the rebuilding route and had refused the drug therapy. So he dragged Peggy down to San Antonio, and for one year they stayed with me. He remained faithful to his program and felt wonderful. His blood work improved dramatically. He got involved in exercise programs and began attending a "church group" which focused on spiritual healing. He was off and running.

Peggy remained in her reclusive state. She reluctantly did a small portion of her program and we had to fuss at her constantly for that. She was locked in a drama, from which, for all my pleadings and prayers, she never emerged. Soon she missed her grandchildren, and since she was convinced that she would die anyway, she went home to spend time with them.

I must say, she was "as a sheep led to the slaughter." She never so much as glanced in another direction. As she became weaker and thinner and balder, Ray became more and more depressed. He felt guilty that she was sick. He didn't want to live without her. Soon he abandoned his program and also sank into despair. With his resolve weakened, he reluctantly began taking the drugs offered him. He finally began to exhibit signs of the disease and he became increasingly sicker and weaker.

Since Peggy was so anemic with the drugs, they never offered them to her again. So now the tables turned. Ray was in an awful state and Peg's blood work was getting healthier. Actually, ever since that bout in the hospital with the pneumonia, and I read to her *The Art of Spiritual Healing,* her blood work steadily improved. Clinically speaking she looked good; none of the usual symptoms of the disease appeared, ever again.

Still she continued to decline and remained in her depressive state. She refused to eat, talk or get out of bed. I left the clinic every Thursday afternoon and flew out to San Francisco to take care of them through the weekends. By now I had despaired of ever seeing the situation change. I knew that by standing for the truth, and through prayer, I could hold the line for them just so long. But there would need to be a change in their own consciousness, a leaving behind of more than they could or would, and an embracing of that which they never did understand.

It is difficult to turn away from the dragons, when you never learned to deal with the monkeys first.

By now both of them were in twin beds in their room. We pushed the beds close together so they could hold hands. Ray was too sick to eat much. He got thinner and sank deeper into a dying state. Peggy on the other hand, simply refused to live. While her spirit was shut to life, her blood work continued to improve. At this point all I could do was crawl into bed with her and hold her and tell her what a wonderful sister she was. Actually, what a wonderful person she was. As children, we started out in hell. Somehow she managed, not only to lift herself up out of it all, but to drag me with her. I'm grateful that I finally stopped nagging her and was able to spend some time telling her how much she meant to all of us.

It was as if each one was waiting for the other to die first. Neither wanted to leave the other behind. Ray died first and two days later my precious sister followed him. While waiting for him she dropped to forty pounds. It was determined that Peggy died, not from AIDS, but from starvation and a broken spirit. She had not one physical symptom of the disease.

Her belief took her. Her expectation. That which she held in the image of her mind. Mass mesmerism to an inordinate attraction to misery.

CHAPTER NINETEEN

JUDGE
RIGHTEOUS
JUDGMENT

Whanat exactly is disease? Is it a solid entity? Something very tangible and substantial? Or is it, as darkness is merely the absence of light, simply the absence of order and harmony? If so, dis-ease could be classified as any interruption in any area of our lives—anything that produces confusion, disorder, and chaos, whatever and wherever there is a loss of order. Then we could focus on reestablishing the God-intended order and harmony into any given situation, thereby removing the dis-ease. This would eliminate the very futile practice of hitting disease head-on, giving it such a gigantic amount of power in our lives, and then wondering why it is ruling over us, to our destruction.

Instead of directing our focus on our body if we are sick, or on our jobs if our careers are stagnating, or on whatever seems to be the area of disorder, we need to look in the direction of our thoughts.

Is peace ruling all our affairs? Do we have a peaceful feeling concerning our relationship with God? Do we feel peaceful in our relationships at home? With our parents? Are we at peace with all our fellow workers and neighbors? What about on the highway or at the grocery store? Most of all, are we at peace with ourselves?

Do we realize the image that God holds about each one of us? Are we able to feel about ourselves and others what He knows and feels about each one of us? Do we know what God "sees" concerning us? Or do we believe that He judges as we judge, strictly according to what our eyes see, our ears hear, our check book declares or what our bodies feel?

> And the spirit of the Lord shall rest upon him, the spirit of wisdom and understanding, the spirit of knowledge and the fear of the Lord, . . . And He shall not judge after the sight of his eyes neither reprove after the hearing of his ears but with righteousness shall he judge the poor, and reprove with equity for the meek of the earth: . . . For the earth shall be full of the knowledge of the Lord, as the waters cover the sea.
>
> ISAIAH 11

What I'm getting at is this . . . since God describes Himself as Divine Love, and we, being made in the likeness of that Being, must conclude that this Love is the true substance of our very being. If we are "choking down" the flow of that Love in any area of our lives, we are blocking the life-giving energy that is required to flow through us to maintain the wholeness and health of our bodies.

We can, by reestablishing the flow of Love, actually bring our lives back into Divine Order and once again experience the health of our bodies. Our bodies, our finances, our jobs, our homes and families are all physical expressions of the thoughts that we embrace on a daily basis. Change the thoughts and we change the physical manifestations of our lives.

Probably the most common theme throughout the Scriptures is the idea of the Mercy of God and Its dynamic influence in the lives of those who recognize it. The only prerequisite to experiencing this ever-present Mercy is that we have the same mercy for others as we desire for ourselves. If we hold hard judgments towards anyone, regardless of how *right* we may think we are, we block the flow of Divine Love in and through our lives and bodies.

The key to being able to do this, in the face of sometimes horrible events and frightening experiences, is this understanding: Absolute Divine Love holds this judgment towards all of Its creation, "that God made us in His image and likeness and nothing can ever alter that fact of our true existence." We do not know that, and therefore, take on various and strange ideas of ourselves, which causes us to act in various, strange ways. But the absolute is still the absolute. The way to see this in ourselves is to see it in others.

There were two patients during my twenty-five years

of clinic practice that demonstrated this principle in the most dramatic way.

Early on I met a young woman whom I will call Betty. She came from a wealthy and prominent family; her mother was well known among the "religious" circles around town. I cannot remember what first brought her to the clinic. It wasn't very serious and she didn't stay long. But several years later she returned, now divorced and living with her toddler son at her mother and father's house. She had just returned from one of the clinics across the border with a diagnosis of metastatic breast cancer and with a prognosis of only a few weeks left to live. She looked every bit as though she would fulfill that prophecy. She was thin and weak and had a tumor the size of an orange protruding out from her breastbone. She was not interested in the program, only that I would continue her daily IV treatments from Mexico for the relief of pain. I agreed to help her any way I could. So her mother brought her to the clinic everyday for me to start her IV drip. When it was over, she would stumble out to the car and head back home. This went on for about ten days or so. Because a weekend was coming, and I lived almost an hour from my clinic, her mother agreed to bring her out to my home for her treatments.

My sister and brother-in-law were visiting (a year before they became ill) and I remember that Betty was so weak that Ray had to carry her into the house. Her veins were collapsing and I was having trouble getting the drip started, so I asked everyone to leave the room so that I could concentrate better. I knelt down in front of her legs, got the IV going, and decided to stay there and hold it steady while the solution was going in. We never spoke a word. She sat with her eyes shut and her head resting on the back of the reclining chair. I heard her mutter something like, "Father, I am not far from your kingdom, now."

I looked at her pathetic form, with all the lumps and bumps coming out, thin and wasted with the ravages of disease. I hated what I saw. I felt the same mixture of rage and helplessness which was all too familiar to me. In desperation, I too, silently prayed. All I remember saying was, "I know I have nothing to offer her. And I also know that Your Love is too pure to allow such a thing to exist. But because of what I see, I do not know how to reconcile this." After the solution was in, Ray carried her back to her car and they drove away.

The next day when she came in I was too busy at the clinic to stop, so I asked someone else to attend to her for me. I remembered feeling something different with her, but I never stopped long enough to think about it again. The following day the same thing happened. Again, I noticed a difference; and again, I never slowed down long enough to investigate it. On the third day, as she was walking past me I grabbed her arm and asked, "Are you healed?" She smiled and said, "Yes." With that she produced CAT scans, MRI's, and blood studies all showing a normal, albeit rather thin, healthy young woman. The tumor in front of her chest was gone. She said that she began to feel better as soon as she left my house that past weekend. She knew that God had healed her. I knew something infinitely more.

I knew that God was honoring my knowing and declaring His Love and Goodness, in spite of what my eyes were seeing and my experience was saying. I knew He was saying, "Yes, that is Who I am. And this is what I know her to be." I was beyond ecstatic. For the healing, yes. But most of all for the unquestioned revealing of the truth concerning God and man. Now, without a doubt, I knew that this understanding was the "Path of Life", the Principle of Life. This then, is the position we are to take, regardless of the circumstances or events.

She actually regained all her strength immediately. So I didn't see much of her after that. There was one incident that happened, though, that did rather disturb me. She had told me earlier that she and her mother were suing her ex-husband for child custody. She was determined not to let him even have visitation rights. She was really into this lawsuit, and the hate and agitation that always accompanies that type of activity. I remember saying to her that I felt that she was heading for disaster if she continued. She became very angry with me for saying that, went right to the phone and called her mother. They whispered for awhile, then she left. I never saw her again. Her evident lack of mercy, when she, herself, had received such mercy from God, was truly a concern to me.

One year later her cancer came back. And though I never got a chance to visit with her again, I knew in my heart what had happened. Betty did die, but in my way of thinking, not from the disease. Through her unwillingness to see her ex-husband in the same light that God saw her, she choked down the flow of the Spirit of Life through her being. And where there once was light and Life, there remained only darkness and death.

Another similar incident happened only a few years ago.

I met a gentleman and his wife after he had already been through radiation for cancer in his spine. It was undaunted by the radiation treatment. Now it had spread to many areas of his bones. Even his right arm was broken from the presence of this disease. He had lost 76 pounds already. After I had interviewed them, they were going back to their home state to pack up their lives and move to this area, to be treated at the clinic. When they walked out of the door, I remember saying to my associate that I wondered if he would even be able to stay alive long enough for them to return. But they did make it back and started on the program immediately.

I really knew nothing about the man, except that he owned his own business and was also carrying quite a lot of anger against his doctor. The story goes that two years prior he went in to have a mole removed and was to be called if there was a problem with the pathology results. When he did not hear from his doctor he assumed that all was in order. A year later he began experiencing pain in his lower spine. It was then discovered that the mole had been malignant and now had spread to all parts of his body. They told me that they were suing this doctor and thought that I would certainly realize their right to do so.

This time, remembering my experience with Betty years before, I took a much stronger stand. I actually read a story to them from Matthew, Chapter 18, in the New Testament, where a king had ordered everyone in his kingdom to pay all their debts owed to him. His servants dragged a man into the presence of the king, crying and begging and pleading for the king to forgive him his debt, because he had no money to pay him. The king had mercy on the man and forgave him his debt and sent him away, a free man. Outside of the palace, the man found another man who owed him much less money than had been forgiven him. He took him by the throat and demanded that he pay. The second man also begged and pleaded to be forgiven his debt, but the first man would not yield. Now the servants to the king saw all that this man had done and went and told the king. The king was furious and called for the man to return to him. He said to him, "I forgave you your debt to me, but you showed no mercy to your brother, and refused to forgive him his debt. You will be thrown into jail until you pay me all that you owe me."

When I finished reading this the patient and his wife were both crying and asked, "What are we to do?" I told them to forgive their doctor and stop the lawsuit immediately. I told them that it was within the realm of human fallibility to make a mistake. And that his life was never in the hands of the doctor anyway, but in the hands of God. It would be idolatry to put a man in the place of God like that.

The story must have impacted them, because they did stop the lawsuit. He went on to become stronger and regain his weight. In four months he was back to his original weight and the pain was gone. When he went for a repeat check-up, with all the scans and tests available, it was determined that the cancer was gone. Even the bones were restored.

For nearly two years he stayed strong and healthy. He built a new home for himself and his wife and we all became great friends. Soon though, the pain returned in his back. The tests showed a return of the cancer and despite all the efforts that we could employ, he also died, seemingly from the cancer. I was asked to officiate at his funeral. That day I learned that, four months earlier, an attorney from his hometown called him and convinced him and his wife to open the lawsuit again. Once again, the free flow of Divine Love, which is also our Life, was choked down by a refusal to see our brothers in the light of God...and therefore, withhold our gift of mercy and life from them. We all do it and we all suffer because of it. It is the law of sowing and reaping, cause and effect. A week before he died, a check from the insurance company came in the mail.

By contrast, a patient came to us from California with a mammogram report of "widely diffuse intraductal carcinoma of the right breast." This particular type of cancer has a reputation of being the most vicious and aggressive of all the various types of breast cancer.

I must attempt to describe Janet to you. She wasn't at the clinic one week before she knew everybody's name and what type of cookies each one liked the most, patient and employee alike. She stayed up nights and baked, and daily arrived with snacks and treats for everyone. Each person had his own program to follow, which was often different from the others, so Janet also found out what they were allowed to eat, and what not, and always made the cookies and cakes according to each specific need. I am talking about maybe forty or fifty people here! She never deviated from her own program, and never complained. Though she was in terrific pain, no one would have known it from watching her. As a matter of fact, although she was here a total of ten months, almost none of the other patients knew why she was a patient, which is a rare thing at any clinic. Throughout the entire ordeal, Janet remained loving and giving and totally un-focused on herself. She refused to dwell on her situation, choosing rather to spend the time meeting the needs of those around her. This was not a new thought to Janet. I have known her most of my life and have never known her to be otherwise. She is loved and cherished by all that know her. Love is not simply a focus with her, but a way of life.

The spiritual truth to be known here is this. There are those who are entrenched in the idea that we must reach out to God if we are going to find Him at all. We must 'choose' Him and follow certain doctrines and beliefs, if we are to receive anything at all from Him. We must offer multitudes of prayers, and ask scores of peoples to also pray for us. In short, we must "do" our part.

The contradiction here is that Janet was an agnostic. She didn't deny God, but didn't acknowledge Him, either. She really didn't know and really never seemed to care. And yet, you can readily see how Divine Love freely flowed through her and how It met her need, in spite of her apparent disinterest in spirituality. Once, and only once, did she ever mention God in a conversation with me. She said that she would feel like a hypocrite to ask God for help when she had ignored Him all these years. This was my answer to her: "If you spent your whole life never noticing the birds singing, though they sang for you everyday, and one day after so many years, you finally did notice them, do you think that they would fold their wings together, throw their little heads up in the air and refuse to sing for you, in anger and protest against the many years you ignored them? The same is true of God, Who, out from His own Being, brought forth the birds." Just as the singing of the birds is an impersonal activity, brought forth from their own nature; so also, is the activity of Divine Love and Life. It brings all that comes into Its Presence into Divine Order. It acts out from Its own Nature, not in response to us. We can only yield to Its Presence. By exercising Love, Janet did this, without even knowing it.

Once again, we are dealing with Mercy and ever-present Divine Love, not our own efforts of righteousness. Once the flow is opened, everything in Its path is set in Divine Order. Janet, knowing nothing of 'the Path', simply kept the flow open by loving. You see, Janet didn't know God, but God knew Janet. And He saw in her His own completion. Though she never knew Him by name, she was a living, breathing expression of Divine Love, with absolutely nothing to obstruct Its flow.

A clear definition of Love then, is not an emotion, as we have been led to believe. It is a choice. A choice to see and know and realize that, no matter how extreme and extensive the appearance may be to the contrary, behind the veil of appearances stands the Glory of the Creator, God in all of His Beauty and Order and Harmony.

> The earth is the Lord's, and the fullness thereof; the world, and they that dwell therein.
>
> PSALMS

> For of Him, and through Him, and to Him, are all things.
>
> ROMANS

> He is the true Light that lighteth every man that cometh into the world.
>
> JOHN

So, as we choose mercy in our vision of others, we restore the flow of Divine Love within ourselves. Remove the *dis-ease,* and it will follow that the *physical problem* is resolved.

CHAPTER TWENTY

WHAT IS LIFE?

We have all found ourselves actors and actresses in the drama of life as we have defined it so far. We have *seen* or interpreted life purely from what we have been educated to believe is true. Do we believe it because we see it, or do we see it because we first believed it to be true?

At any rate, there is God's vision of Life as He formed it from His imagination and then there is man's way of seeing things. One brings the glories of life and the other, all the confusion that we presently live in. The trick here is to be willing to let go of the one and to search out the other. Instead of holding in thought the well-worn concept of life, let's try a new one and see if the effort of planting this seed will bring forth a harvest of good experiences in our lives.

As we have seen the wondrous healings at the clinic

for so many years by cleansing the body of accumulated environmental toxins, so now let us take this obviously successful concept into the realm of the mind and by the "renewing of our minds" prove what has truly been given to us by God. "As we have borne the image of the earthy, let us reach out to bear the image of the heavenly." Let us look at and define the image of the heavenly. And while we are doing this, let us keep in mind that it is in this image that we have been formed and given Life.

What is Life? Sounds like a pretty silly question, doesn't it? All of us know what life is, don't we? Or do we?

There was a time when I thought I knew the answer to that question, and on a very superficial level of thought, I did. But as the years went by, and with them so many experiences concerning what we call "life and death" issues, I had to look at my understanding of life. I had to examine my prevailing thoughts and begin to question the legitimacy of them. Soon the borders and limitations began to expand and give way to an understanding—and the understanding to an experience of such wonder and such clarity! With this, my whole view, my whole perception, my approach to disease and the elimination of it, had to change. Actually, my approach to the whole experience called life itself changed.

We, of course, define life in terms of being born, growing, maturing, aging and dying. Dying is referred to as the end of life, birth is the beginning. All the scrambling in the middle is the total experience called *my life*. With this in view, we must make the best possible experience out of it all. "Life is short." "We get out of life what we put into it." "Survival of the fittest."

Around every turn we are told to get out there and make it happen! "Do it before it's done to you." Become the *fittest* or become the victim of the *fittest*. Life becomes a race to the finish line, and when we get there we fight not to cross it. The journey is fast, laborious, exhausting, scary, uncertain and oftentimes ruthless.

We become competitive because we judge the success of our efforts against the success of others. Our view of success is how long we lasted in the race, how far we got by way of worldly accomplishments, and how much we acquired along the way. We are the "sun" of our life, and we are responsible to keep all the props rotating around us in perfect harmony, at all times. We are responsible to make "it" happen. It is our effort, our sweat. We carry around the burden of our life. If we do well by these standards, we are bloated with self-importance. If we do mediocre by these standards, we are filled with self-condemnation and regrets. Both are equally as destructive.

Is there any wonder that there is dis-ease as a result? Is there any wonder we hide away in pills, alcohol, and food? Is it any wonder we hide away in the lives of others, as in soap operas, sports, movies, TV, and novels? Is it any wonder we lack the courage to face life as thus defined?

We are at the center of our interpretation of life. Therefore, we might address this view of life more aggressively and become the "bully on the block." We might choose to accumulate letters behind our name to better secure our rather tentative positions. We might demand respect through the acquisition of wealth or position, houses or lands. We might become cynical and judgmental of others to divert attention away from our own inadequacies. Any way we look at it, it is a "no win" situation. No matter how we run the race, from the time we explode from the starting line until the end of the race, we are personally responsible and therefore completely exhausted. Definitely dis-eased!

Might I make the suggestion that disease can be a speed bump along the way? At best. Or an escape, at worst. But certainly it is a result of such an all-consuming thought process. If we approach life in this manner, as we all have been taught to do, we will realize one day—when we hit a speed bump or when we get to the end of it—that we missed it altogether.

I remember in my late teens, when I was a student nurse and later a practicing nurse, watching scores of people die. It was evident early on that there were two distinctly different scenarios going on, and each individual fell into one or the other. On one hand, there were those who fought and resisted the process, or those who simply acquiesced in submissive depression. They were by far the majority. On the other hand there were those who had such a serenity about them, such an expression of peace it could not be denied. They clearly knew something that I didn't know! I used to wonder about it all. I mentioned it to others along the way, hoping for some enlightenment, but received none. One thing was clear—most people missed something that very few really got.

What I have been describing is the general worldview, or interpretation, of life. I believe that it carries with it some definite consequences and one of these is disease. Disease of the body, mind and spirit. Other consequences might be the fracturing of families, broken homes and hearts. Other consequences might be wars, accidents, poverty and really any other picture of misery that we can conjure up in our imagination. I believe that all sadness and sorrow is a result of the type of mind set that the world-thought embraces as reality.

I believe that since misery is so prevalent, we have come to accept it as part of life—a necessity of life. Instead of challenging it, we accept it, then try to find reasons why it exists. If disease is so necessary, if there is no way around it, then why do we spend so much time, effort and finances trying to defeat it? We defeat one disease only for ten more to arise.

CHAPTER TWENTY-ONE

LIFE IS GOD—
GOD IS LIFE

Finally, one day the simple understanding came, so gently that I thought I had known it my whole life. God is Life. God is the only Life that there is. God does not give us life. God is our Life. There is only One Life. Not many, but One. That One Life expresses Itself as the whole of creation, including us. We are not as we thought we were. Everything is an expression of God, of Life. Life is eternal. It has no beginning, no ending. That is why the Bible says that we were "in Him" before the world was. To be "in Him" is to be in this one Life.

Life is not an event, it is a Person. An expression of that Person. Life does not start with our birth, It does not end with our death and It does not have Its origin within our body. We live in Life. Life does not live within us. It flows through us, as It does all of creation.

We don't need to check it out by looking at our blood or x-rays or temperature. We need to look outside of the body. We need to look away from the body. We have been looking in the wrong direction. If we want to know the condition of our life, we must look at this Eternal, endless Life. We cannot *attain* to Life. This is critical. We have only to recognize that Life is God, already whole, complete, perfect and breathtakingly beautiful. And we exist as expressions of that Life, breathtakingly beautiful.

We have been sadly mistaken about our image of ourselves. We see ourselves as incomplete and pitiful and sinful and somehow dirty. We have been looking through a veil. And we have been living our lives out from the rubble of such a vision. Our expectation has been according to our "sense of unworthiness."

We must immerse ourselves in the vision that this Life holds about us. We must gain the sense of completeness, of worthiness, of wholeness. If we FEEL whole, healthy, strong and full of the glory of Life, believe me, we will manifest that and only that.

Jesus said that to gain Life, we must first be willing to lose our (sense of) life. He said we must deny our "self life." Any sense of a self-life must be turned away from, and the SENSE of, or FEELING of Life "outside of ourselves" must be embraced. St. Paul said, " It is no longer I that liveth." But this new awareness of Life, so Divine, so radiant, so beautiful, is what liveth. Instead of the old, fearful, limited vision of life within the body, subject to the false demands of the body, now is come Life that daily fills our hearts with strength, with love and laughter. Now we turn away from the pathetic props of old, the rubber crutches of the old life vision, and we gladly immerse ourselves in the new understanding.

Now we cease to reach out to an illusive God of many demands in order to attain righteousness. Now we receive and embrace Righteousness AS our very life. We have no life to offer. There is only Eternal, Divine Life living out Its own righteousness AS us.

We don't have to choose It. It has chosen us. The only requirement from us is that we willingly receive It. We receive It by opening our minds and hearts to Its presence, much like we receive air into our lungs by breathing it in. We never question that there is air all about us, even though we don't see it. It does not force its way into our lungs, we must take it in. Did we "earn" the air? Were we good enough? Or is the only requirement that we take it in? If we are standing in the shade and we're cold, we can simply move over to where the sun is shining. The warmth of the sun is always there, only we must move into it. "The sun rises on the good and evil alike. The rain falls on the just and the unjust alike." What does this mean? It means simply this: This Life is poured out—period. It is not earned. It cannot be earned. It only sees Itself, pure and holy. And It sees us, as Itself. So it sees "in us" Its own Worth, always.

Now we see ourselves and others according to our learned belief, and we act out from that belief. But the vision of God is according to HIS OWN existence. He did not make multitudes of lives. There is only one Life, but multitudes of expressions of that One Life. From the trees, the stars, the insects, and animals, to us.

If we appear sick or sad or limited in any way, we are living out a belief. We are "buying into" a picture, on the canvas of our mind, that has been painted and drawn by thousands of words spoken in fear and ignorance throughout a lifetime. But long ago, before time was, a Word was spoken by the Eternal Mind. "And without that Word was not anything made that was made. All things were made by the Word. And that Word was the Life and the Light of man."

We are a result of that Word. Nothing, not even the convoluted words of ignorance, not centuries of misunderstanding and confusion, not that which is misbelieved, not that which is seen by minds darkened behind the veil of "unknowing," nothing, absolutely nothing can ever, nor has ever, changed that Word.

It is not our responsibility to "be" the image and likeness of God. We did not choose God. God chose us. We have no reason to try to "be" anything. We have only to yield, to relax, to surrender our efforts and "receive" that which already is.

CHAPTER TWENTY-TWO

CHALLENGING PREVAILING RELIGIOUS THOUGHT

Although they are quick to deny this, I have found that most people believe that God is in some way responsible for their suffering. Some believe that they are being punished for past or present behavior by a Supreme Being, located outside of themselves, to whom they are accountable. They believe this on one hand, but then scramble around trying to find someone who can get them out of their situation—that God Himself put them in. Now, if we hold the thought that God has decreed this suffering for us, why do we search out a mere man to change our circumstances?

Others believe that God "certainly couldn't do such a thing. He only ALLOWS it to happen to you." As a matter of fact, I have seen disease so ugly, so horrible, so vicious in its appearance, that I would be loath to serve a God who could even devise such horror, or would use it to achieve some end result. What kind of a malicious mind could fabricate such suffering? If a man were to do such to another man, we would immediately search him out and eliminate him from the earth. But we attribute to Him, Who made the earth and all the beauty in it, to be capable of such horror. He, Who counts the very hairs of your head. "Eyes have not seen, nor have ears heard, neither has entered into the heart of man, all that God has prepared for them, who cling to Him." Who cling to Him in Truth and Understanding.

Realizing such a contradiction of thought, we say that God is Love and therefore could not do such to his beloved creation. How are we to reconcile such confusion?

On one hand, we have man, made in the image of a perfect Creator. Perfect means flawless. Flawless includes incapable of error. We are created in that same image; we are "His workmanship, created unto perfection, made in the image and LIKENESS of God." That is our nature, our being.

But, we're told that man was born with the capacity to turn away from his own nature. To choose against his own God-given nature, to his own destruction. Now can we find any other created being that is capable of turning away from its own nature? And thus self-destruct? How could God be described with such confusion and contradiction? And so we go on.

Then, according to the general teaching, after we are created unto such convoluted thought, we are punished, by the very same Creator that assigned us so. But not really by Him, they say, because "God is Love." But by a force of evil, so terrible in its appearance, and yet created by this Love, which punishes us with such permanence and destruction.

Now why am I going on and on like this? Why is this so important to me as to put my head on the religious chopping block by challenging these widespread doctrines?

Just this: People are dying. People are agonizing with pain that won't be relieved. People are suffering unspeakable horrors. Unless you've been in medicine or involved in health care in some way, you cannot imagine what I'm saying. Mental depression and anxiety are running rampant throughout the world. And it is all so unnecessary. We as a human race accept it all because we believe we somehow deserve it. Somewhere we messed up. We believe we are responsible to do better because we have been told that from the beginning—and we messed up. Now we must suffer the consequences.

How many hundreds of times have I watched and listened to the cries and confusion of my patients? "What have I done? What could I have done better? What (magic) prayer can I offer to stop this misery? Where, in my personal responsibility to live life righteously, did I fail?" Or, " If I get more and more people to pray for me, then maybe my suffering will be relieved. Maybe God will hear if a lot of people pray. Maybe that will cause Him to have mercy and change His mind."

I listen and I feel my gut wrenching within me. It is all so unnecessary. Every pastor in the country will have to admit that the same fate befalls those with religious convictions as well as those who have none. We're dying like flies, or we're living in fear of death. There's not much difference, really. But there is a way out of this.

There is a way out. But there is a prerequisite to understanding the way out. Jesus said it best when He said, "You cannot put new wine in old wineskins." We must first be willing to empty out of our mind the old thoughts, the contradictions, and the confusion that we have inadvertently absorbed. The definition of the word repent is: "To change one's mind. To turn towards another direction." If we desire truth, more than the false security of the old landmarks, then we must *repent* of what we have believed and explore on. "Repent, for the Kingdom of Heaven is at hand." When we turn from the old, and wait to humbly embrace the new, the Kingdom of "wholeness, joy, health, fulfillment and peace" will be at hand.

Basically, I am aware that the things I say here are not mainstream thought or belief. But after looking at the chaos and confusion in the lives and health of the world today, isn't it time to humbly turn away from our cherished beliefs? Isn't it time to reach out to a True and Loving Creator, Who is holding out the Light of pure truth and understanding, illuminating the path before us, that we might enjoy Life, as was always intended?

What is LIFE? What we have been calling life, has turned to be death to us. So with weary arms and heavy hearts, we sigh and gladly lay down our efforts and our misunderstandings. We lay them at the feet of true Mercy and Divine Love and wait for enlightenment and understanding that will be to us, Life.

CHAPTER TWENTY-THREE

REMOVING
THE VEIL

Many years ago I stumbled across a Scripture in Isaiah in the Old Testament which said, "The Lord would destroy a covering that was cast over all people, and the veil that is spread over all nations." And when this veil, or covering, was removed, He would ". . . swallow up death in victory and the Lord, God, would wipe away tears from all faces." I then read a corresponding Scripture in the book of Revelation in the New Testament, that promised a wiping away of tears, sorrow, suffering, and disease and death. When I read this, it arrested my thought. I suddenly realized that there was a veil, a covering that covered all people. It covered their faces, their vision, their understanding and their ability to know. And when that veil was removed, there would be no more suffering and sadness. All tears would be wiped away. All disease and misery would be gone from our experience. Think of a world without pain or sickness or tears!

This would occur, not when we were proven to have earned it. Not when we were *good* enough. Not when medical science discovered another cure for another disease, leaving another several hundred diseases yet to be healed. Not when we understood dietary laws and became perfectly compliant to them. Not when all the *bad* people in the world were finally punished, leaving the "righteous" to inherit the wonders of creation. But this promise would appear only when this veil was removed. So the problem was the veil. Not the disease. Not us. Not God. Not our heredity. Not our cholesterol. But the problem was that we were blinded to what was true, what was real, by the presence of a covering. The problem was the covering, the veil. Just remove the veil and the problem goes. In comes the light of truth, and out goes the darkness of chaos and confusion.

At that moment, I turned away from seeing disease as having any other origin. I stopped seeing suffering as having any other origin. I stopped seeing human misery as having any other origin, except a lack of light, a lack of understanding. Somehow, what we have clung to as the truth of God, of life, of our relationship to Life, and therefore to God, was a convoluted, distorted vision from peering through a veil in front of our eyes.

Our vision was in question here, not our bodies. What happened to our bodies was a result of what we *saw*. And what we saw was what we came to believe was true. What we believed was true was what we expected. What we expected was what we got. Perception bccame reality.

Then, while musing over these thoughts for what seemed like months, I found a Scripture that declared that the veil was already removed *in Christ*. Was already removed! Now there was absolutely no reason for a continuation of suffering, of disease. So, what was this veil? And what does *in Christ* really mean? Many people say that they are *in Christ,* and they are still suffering and dying of the same diseases that other people are afflicted with. What does it really mean?

I want to tell the story that began to answer these questions. The experience that challenged my entire perspective of Life, of God, and of my responsibility in it all. It took me years and years to get over this event. Needless to say, when I finally emerged, everything I had believed had changed. Before, I thought that I knew about Life, about God. Now I knew Life as God.

In 1982, I met a wonderful, young girl, who had breast cancer. Her name was Margaret. She and her husband and three children moved from Alaska to my home and lived there for two years while she remained on the "program" at the clinic. Her situation, her physical care, the care of her young children, all took a tremendous amount of focus and literally consumed our lives. Prayer for her was continual. I threw all my hope, emotionally, into her recovery. This was quite early on, during the time I was struggling with so many questions about Life and God and what it was really all about. I prayed every prayer, read every Scripture, believed every Word. Although I had long before abandoned the world's view of the "race" called Life, and I had lost all interest in what seemed to be the foolish aspirations of that race, still I was running a race of my own. It was a Spiritual race, to who-knew-where. I think I believed that if I prayed enough, read enough, believed enough, and agonized over my patients enough, that would please God and He would then heal them. What a dreadful vision of a dreadful God.

But no matter my efforts, she was not getting well. I could feel my props, shaky as they were, falling out from under me. I simply could not give more or do more. All my believing, all my efforts were to no avail. It was the single most painful spiritual experience I ever had. Everything I had been told about God was being challenged. Everything was falling apart and I was free falling through the air with nothing to hold onto. I wanted so badly to understand, but understand what?

A few weeks before she died, I had a very explicit and detailed dream. The kind you never forget. This was my dream: I was one of several hundred people who were all dressed in white "sweats," running a race, hard and fast. I was so proud of myself because I was among those who were out in front. I knew I would get to the finish line before most. Suddenly, there was some commotion directly in front of me. I couldn't tell exactly what was going on at first, but soon it became apparent that someone had collapsed and was lying in the roadway. Everyone was tripping and jumping over her. No one wanted to break his stride and fall behind. I started to jump over her, myself, but I couldn't do it.

I knew I could never leave her there to be trampled. So I stopped and dragged her off the road into some tall, thick weeds. She was unconscious, so I put her head on my lap and sat and watched the other runners go by. My heart was sad to realize that I was no longer in the race. I could never win now. All my efforts were for nothing. Also, at the same time, I was embarrassed that I was entertaining such selfish thoughts. Finally night came, and the last of the runners had passed us by. I was sitting, looking at the stars, when suddenly she became a male, and with the softest, tenderest voice, He said, "Don't worry, Michele. You have not lost the race. Learn this. The race is not to the swift, nor the battle to the strong, but to them who show mercy. To them, the race is already won. This is not Margaret that you have been caring for, but Me."

It took me a long time to assimilate all that was in that dream. It would be many years and many more experiences before I would be able to grasp all that the dream contained.

Gradually, I began the long process of letting go of a "false sense of responsibility," for one thing. I stopped focusing on the diseases, as though they were the real problem. I realized that behind the veil of mortality was "the Christ," in every person I met, in every patient I saw. I realized that there was no race to be run, nothing to be gained at all by the exercise of human effort. If I looked deep beyond the human circumstances and the situation presented to me, I would see the *completeness and wholeness* already present that I thought I had to work so hard to create.

Above all else, I learned what is really required of us as we move in and among those we encounter. And that is, of course, to show mercy. Mercy is kindness, tenderness and gentleness, even to the "undeserved." Mercy generally involves some degree of self-sacrifice. But above that, mercy is to choose to see *through* their image of themselves, whether it is sickness, or human ugliness of any kind, and to see "Christ."

Christ is a term used for ". . . the visible expression of the invisible God." This is how God, Eternal Love and Life, actually deals with us all. He sees beyond our sometimes poor, pathetic image of ourselves and sees His own Nature, His own Eternal, unchangeable Selfhood, in us.

It was a long and difficult task for me to be able to turn away from what I had been taught to believe. To be free of the old vision, to be able to grasp the new. I think I wanted to understand more than I wanted to breathe. At the same time, I seemed to fight the new from coming. I knew that I didn't want to waste any more time wandering around the desert of dry doctrines, finding the bones of those who had wandered before me.

But where to go for a pure understanding? Obviously, I knew that I must go nowhere. I must trust that God had led me this far. No one in their right mind would spend this much time and effort searching out what would appear to be an impossible journey, except that God was leading them.

So, every morning, I would walk for two hours and enjoy the wonders of Life as they appeared to me and I would pray and wait for the veil to be lifted and for Truth to reveal itself. Actually, one day an unusual thing happened to me. It was a simple, yet endearing encouragement from God along the way.

I used to have an invisible eraser and I would daily use it to erase from my mind everything that had cluttered it. Then I would hand the chalk to the "Spirit of Truth" and tell Him to write the true understanding, the true picture on the "canvas of my mind." I went through this little routine every day for years. This particular day I was feeling very frustrated. I prayed, "I wish I could spend just one day with the wisest man ever to live, so that all my questions could be finally answered." Even as I said it I laughed at myself. I knew that I already spent every day with the Wisest Man ever to live, and that He was teaching me and would continue to do so throughout eternity.

As these thoughts were going on in my mind, I suddenly heard a rustle in the trees and leaves next to the narrow country road where I was walking. I looked over to see a doe climb up onto the road and walk over towards me. To my amazement, she began to walk beside me. Now I don't need to say that deer do not walk up to humans and stroll along with them, do I? At first I was afraid to breathe. I was afraid to break my stride in any way and frighten her away. We walked for about a mile, side by side, and I decided to try something. I deliberately walked to the other side of the road to see what she would do. She right away crossed over behind me and began walking next to me on the other side. I still had one more test I felt compelled to try. I knew that in a few hundred yards I would have to turn left onto my street. I thought, "If she turns with me, I will know that I am walking with the 'Wisest Man ever to live,' who has chosen to appear as this gentle doe." And so she did. Not only that, but she followed me right up to my house and stood in the driveway while I went in to get ready for work. When I came out, she was gone. It was a simple little, "I know this is taking a long time, but I'm still with you. Hang on!"

CHAPTER TWENTY-FOUR

THE WONDER OF LIFE
MAINTAINED IN DIVINE ORDER

There are, in my mind, two main attributes of God that really define Him. They describe His Life, and therefore, our Life, as well as the Life and Substance of all creation. I believe that the mystery of Life, and all the issues of Life, are wrapped up in the understanding of these two characteristics of God.

One, we have discussed as Divine Love. This, again, is the Mercy and judgment of God, whereby He sees past the veil of mortal thinking and reasoning into the beauty and perfection that constitutes our true being.

The second characteristic of God that enables us to enjoy the wonders of Life, free from the misery of pain and disease—even free of the experiences of accidents and mishaps—would be Divine Order. It is this attribute of Life that holds all of creation intact.

The basic foundational philosophy of the clinic was established through the understanding of the unchangeable order of God. Once I *saw* it and began to really *feel* it, I was better able to understand the origin of the contrasting, or opposite concept, called disease. This understanding then lifted me out from the realm of healing, being a "hit or miss" experience, to an absolute Spiritual Law. That means that it will be available to every receptive heart, no matter the condition to be healed, simply by accepting it. No more "storming heaven" with repetitive prayers and pleadings. And, as is so often the case, still being left with the prayers unanswered. No more wondering if we have said the 'right' prayer, or made ourselves *worthy* enough. No more rationalizing our failure to receive our healing by accepting the absurd thought that it may not be God's will that we be healed.

Let us then pause and examine this aspect of the nature of God. Divine Life defines Itself as Immutable Order. "I AM the Lord, thy God, I change not." Immutability refers to that quality of Divinity, which is unchangeable, permanent and absolute. If we can agree that that which has created all things is, in fact, immutable, then whatever state we have been created in, is also unchangeable in its nature. That is the spiritual law that transcends all physical causation. We also can agree that this Divine Being is Omnipresent. It fills all space with Its nature and Its influence in that It is also Omnipotent. To define Omnipotence as all-powerful, we must conclude that to be all of anything, there cannot be anything outside of that *allness*.

So now, we have a God Who fills all space with His Presence, His power and the unchangeable, absoluteness of His Being and His thought or Mind. Now we can look at this world and choose to see beauty and order and feel the constancy of a Presence that fills our hearts with such wonder. Now everything we look at, we can interpret through the eyes of this understanding and expectancy. Now truly, "The Earth is the Lord's, and the Fullness thereof." Prior to this understanding of God, as Divine Order, all I was able to see was confusion and chaos. Instead of seeing Life all around me, all I could see was death. Instead of seeing goodness, all I could see was sadness and pain.

For many years I stayed focused on seeing beauty everywhere. I insisted on it, no matter what the evidence to the contrary might be declaring. It became a matter of principle with me. If God was declaring Himself as that which fills all space with Presence and Goodness and Power, then that was that. It was a matter of honoring God now, more than wanting to have some human picture corrected.

Through this *resolve* and with much concentrated practice, I learned to *see* and to *feel* the Presence of Omnipresence, right where disease, confusion and disorder were declaring its right to exist. Much to my amazement, just by that acknowledgment, whatever seemed to be *out of order*, rapidly began to take on the appearance of Divine Order.

I thought about everything being in an unchangeable order. I thought about all of Creation telling us of its perfection and order. The seasons come and go, we can count

on that. The days and nights come and go, we can count on
that. The same constellations that appear in the heavens at
any given month are the same ones that have appeared even
before the Earth was formed. We can count on that also,
without fear of change. The same birds come to my bird-
house each year, on the same date, have the same two sets
of nesting, and leave on the same date each year. We can
pick up any issue of *National Geographic Magazine* and it
will be filled with information about every aspect of nature,
and the order and predictability of each species, plant or
animal, star or planet. There is no phase of life that one can
study that will not appear as a revelation of Divine Order.
There is no career path that one can choose where Divine
Order is not evident.

Without this order, all existence as we know it would
collapse. We depend on this order, and for the most part we
trust it without thought. We realize that even when something out of the ordinary does appear, such as a swarm of
caterpillars, for instance, they have appeared only to balance
out another aspect of nature. It is the wise husbandman who
does not interfere with this Wisdom. All balance, all harmony, is a result of, and under the control of this Divine
Order. Nature balances all things and keeps its own intrinsic order intact. The substance of all nature is Divine Life
and, therefore, is self-sustaining. Infinite Wisdom and
Intelligence is actually revealing Itself AS creation. It is upon
this understanding that we build our hope, because we also
are included in this entire scenario. The true substance of
our being is not flesh and blood, as it would appear, but
Divine Life and Intelligence. This is not to be confused with

human wisdom, which cannot be compared to the Eternal Wisdom of Infinity.

It is important that we realize that the same Life that fills every infinite detail of creation also fills us. It is important that we realize that the same Life that animates every infinite detail of creation also animates us. It is also important that we realize that Life alone is the substance of us. It manifests Its Presence as the order, balance and harmony of our body, as well as our mind. It is the Intelligence of every cell in our being. It is the life of every cell in our being. From this vantage point, we are an Eternal being. We existed before we came into this form, and we will continue to exist as Life after we no longer need this form.

But while we are here, Life is expressing Itself as us. Life is expressing Its harmony in the *well ordered being* of the human body. Life is expressing Its Order in the intricate details of the interdependent workings and structures of the human body. Life is expressing Its Balance in the enzymes, hormones, and perfections of the entire cellular system, assimilation and metabolism. We cannot begin to understand all the immense and infinite details of the workings of our bodies, even if we studied it our entire life.

We must learn to *see* Life in our bodies. We must *see* It flowing through us. We must *see* Life as the very *cause* of our existence, as the source and origin of our beings. Now as we trust Life to bring food to its creatures, to bring the seasons to fruition, to bring the daylight, to bring the night, let us learn to trust Life, the very same Life, to maintain the order of the human body and mind and affairs.

Can we not stop this madness, this hysteria, long

enough to step aside from our human efforts and LET Life flow and prove the immutable, perfect workings of Its own Nature? Without all our "flailing" efforts to keep ourselves one step ahead of the grave, would the whole thing collapse?

Have you ever seen cement poured on the ground and soon a piece of grass, or even a tree, bursts forth from the cement? That is Life, insisting on Its own unchangeable, undeniable, uninterruptable nature to flow, and express Itself. Life will not be denied. Does It really need all our frantic human efforts? Or are our efforts just another obstacle to be overcome by Life?

Can Accidents be Supported by Divine Order?

Concerning accidents and other related disasters, we must apply the same understanding as we do for the health of our bodies. If we are consciously cognizant of the knowledge of this Divine Order as the substance of all that is created, as holding all things intact and if we choose to see the evidence of this everywhere we look, the very knowledge of this would preclude not only the "vulnerable victim" attitude towards disease, but also the same attitude towards accidents and natural disasters, which are not natural at all. Just as we can *rise in thought* into the atmosphere of wholeness concerning our bodies, thereby escaping the vulnerability to disease, so we can also rise in thought into the place where we realize that Divine Order is holding Its creation in the "palm of Its hand." If we insist on the reality of this truism, the fear and expectations of accidents and disasters will also cease to exist to us. If we play the victim to any of it, then we are playing the victim to all of it.

Our family experienced a classic example of this principle several years ago. Once again it concerned my daughter, Lara. From the time she was healed and throughout her entire growing years we teased her about being "accident-prone." She had more mishaps than any other child I knew. Once she fell out of a tree and I really thought that was the end of her. Another time she rode her bike directly in front of an oncoming car, though she was told never to ride on that particular street. Even though she went sailing off the bike, the bike was hurt more than she was. Still another incident was of diving into a shallow pool requiring that I put six stitches in her chin. But the worst accident happened while I was out of town, naturally. I bought a new bicycle for her on her sixth birthday. I foolishly bought it too big for her, thinking that she would be able to grow into it and have it for many years. One day while trying to keep up with the older kids, she went flying down a steep hill and couldn't reach the brakes to stop herself. Off she went over the handlebars and careened down the remainder of the hill on her face. She left half her face and four teeth (two permanent) on the road that day. She was unconscious for two days and it took years to piece her back together again. We used to call her "an accident looking for a place to happen." We thought we were so cute, not realizing the mind-set we were programming into her little heart and expectations. Not realizing it until she was a new driver at sixteen and was involved in four accidents in one year! She was not a careless driver; she was a fearful driver. Her fears preceded her at every turn. I knew we had to address this on a spiritual level. This was not a disciplinary problem.

Together we went back in our minds to every accident that we could think of in which she had been involved. We corrected our words and our thoughts, insisting on the reality of Divine Order as being the unchangeable Presence and substance of each incident, even though at the time of the accidents we were not aware of it, and even though the *evidence* was clearly to the contrary. Right where the accidents were *declaring* the absence of any Eternal Order at all, we knew that behind the veil of that human picture stood the immutable truth of absolute Divine Order. We worked on this for several weeks until Lara was sure she had replaced that "consciousness of accidents" with one of order and protection. She never drove fearfully again. She said she never felt that fear again. And, of course, accidents have been a thing of the past.

CHAPTER TWENTY-FIVE

FROM BEING A VICTIM
TO BEING A BEHOLDER

Our good comes to us by what we *see* more than what we do; by what we *know* deep within us, more than by what we say. While it may be necessary to take human footsteps during the course of a disorder, still the healing and the fulfillment can only come with a change in vision. Without this change in perception, the relief is but transitory. But how does this change take place? What is our responsibility in this activity?

After years of holding a certain mind-set, how are we to make our minds see differently? Do we force it? Do we fake it? Do we exercise extreme will power over our own thoughts? For example, if people have spent their lives feeling unloved, unworthy, and useless, not needed, incapable, unhealthy, poverty bound, or any of the like—are we to say,

"Don't think that thought and it will all go away?" How do we get from here to there?

The answer is simply this: *we surrender.* We lay down our efforts, our strivings, and surrender to the Mind of God which will then operate within our minds to correct the error in thought. If we need health we must stop believing that we must *attain* to health and instead surrender to the fact that the mind of God has *forever* held us in a state of health and wholeness. When through devotion and meditation upon this reality, the *feeling* of the truth enters our hearts, at that point either the situation will change spontaneosly or ways will open up to us that we could never have realized before.

If we need direction, whether it concerns a career, a move, a companion, or a way to handle a certain person or situation—we must stop searching for the right human solution. We must stop listening to the advice of others, and instead surrender to the omniscient (all knowing) Mind of God. We will soon know the right way. The Wisdom of God will direct us. There will be no doubts or hesitations.

By doing this, we are not surrendering to the circumstances. We are not surrendering to the disease. We are learning to look *through* them into the heart of Divine Love. At first (and sometimes for a long time) it may be necessary to just stop, quiet our minds, and ask for the grace to realize the thoughts that lie within the Mind of God concerning any given situation. We may have to insist and stay earnestly with that request, particularly if fear or restlessness is crowding into our minds. Soon though, the perfect image will appear, sometimes in a picture, often with a feeling. It can not be mistaken and it can not be missed when it happens. As we practice this day by day it becomes easier, until all that is necessary is simply to pause and without a word or a prayer the pure image is known.

We must not fail to deal with the everyday situations as they appear, rather than merely *putting up* with them in the hopes that they will just somehow go away. It is in applying the truth to the monkeys that enables us to hold our heads high and walk on without fear at the appearances of the dragons.

The very first time this type of thought process was introduced to me was when my daughters were still babies. As I mentioned earlier, Linda was quite prone to fevers and it was one of those incidents that led me to call on the help of a far wiser and more mature woman than myself. My request was that she accompany me to the doctor's office, but her response was something I never imagined. She said that she would come right over and take me if I would do something while she was on her way. She told me to kneel next to Linda (who was lying on a beanbag on the floor, bright red and burning up with fever) and place my hands on her head and quietly and calmly tell the fever to leave her. Quietly and calmly was certainly the key here. If I remained in the frightened and agitated state which I was in when I called for help, I could not have accomplished this. As long as I was giving the *appearance* such power by my fearful reaction, the problem would remain. I was *playing victim* to the situation, having no idea the power available to me to correct it. At first I thought she was kidding me, but when I learned she was not, I said I would "try it" so long as she still was on her way to get us and go for *real* help if it didn't work. As soon as she hung up, I did exactly what she requested. I found that if I sang a song or two for Linda first, we both would calm down. Within minutes after singing the songs and telling the fever to leave, it was gone. Usually when a fever breaks, the patient begins to perspire profusely, but this she did not do. It simply was not there anymore. When my friend arrived, everything was calm and under control. To say that I was amazed would be an understatement.

From that first and obvious proof that suffering, while it came as a physical entity, did not necessarily need to be dealt with on that level—and that we are not in a helpless state when faced with it—I have continued to follow this understanding. Each difficulty is an opportunity to dive deeper into our hearts and find the wisdom that is always present there. Once that knowledge is gained and we follow its directions, it then has an opportunity to prove its legitimacy by healing the situation. We have ascended higher into our rightful place as sons and daughters of God, no longer victims of world thought and blinded to our true identity. We have then gained ascendancy over the vexing monkeys in our life and are better prepared for the dragons when they appear.

After years of dealing with human suffering and tragedy in one form or another, I have learned to see this phenomena no longer as an actual fact of existence, but more as an uninvited visitor. I have learned to deal with all disruptions in life as something outside of us—something trying to *bully* us into yielding to *its* presence or acknowledging *its* power over us. Anything that would attempt to put us into a state of subservience to the circumstance. This can only happen if we allow it to happen. And we allow it in direct proportion to our lack of understanding as to *who* we are and *why* we are here. It was never intended that we would live in defeat to anything.

Our True Identity Revealed

There are many varied states of consciousness in this experience we call life. Think of the different levels in the atmosphere that surround the earth. We are always being drawn higher and higher, from one into the other and on from there. Each level attained represents a clearer view of life as we progress upward and deeper into the heart of Life Itself. As our understanding becomes clearer and our perceptions change, so do our expectations, and therefore, our experiences. Each new revelation is often proceeded by some type of a human struggle as we are unconsciously letting go of the old to embrace the new. If we understand this process, we will not fear the events that caused the struggle in the first place. We can, with awareness of this, simply smile and walk on, realizing that only a shift in perception is taking place and that, in spite of the threat, nothing has ever—nor can ever—change for us, as long as we refuse to empower it. So long as we know that we are still the *unfoldment of the Divine Life,* revealing Itself, expressing and declaring Itself, with each step we take. The events that clamor for our attention are not as they appear. We will choose to look at the path set before us and walk on, knowing that Divine Mind, seeing through our own mind, will correct the picture and order the events. "And an highway shall be there, and a way, and it shall be called The way of holiness . . . No lion shall be there, nor any ravenous beast shall go up thereon, it shall not be found there; but the redeemed shall walk there." (Isaiah 35)

Finally we will reach the atmosphere of understanding, where we no longer live in a hostile environment, in which we must continually duck the blows and deal with the events. We will find that we are a part of Life; that we walk in it and we talk in it and laugh and love in it. We will see that It surrounds us and blesses us with every good thing. We will recognize every bird that sings and every flower that blooms as being there *for us.* We will feel the smile of Life all around us, enveloping us with a penetrating Love that absolutely excludes any thought of the appearance of evil, in any form. When Jesus said that the kingdom of heaven was within us, and when he said that we should "turn away from our old thoughts (repent) and realize that the kingdom of heaven is at hand," it was not a metaphor, not something that was available only to him. This is the reality that has always been present. This is our true home. Nothing can stop us from entering into it.

We will live *above* the scratching and scrambling of

human pain and struggle and find that Life has always been present with us, always surrounded us, and always loved us, even when we knew it not. We will shun entering into conversations that rehearse the drama of anguish, or the tenacious thought that refuses to let it go. The author, Richard Bach, so aptly describes the process of learning to soar high and above such enslaving thought, in his book, *Jonathan Livingston Seagull*. As his little seagull struggles and practices, learning that he has wings that will take him higher than he ever imagined—far above the flock that chooses to stay earthbound— he too finds an existence bursting with the joy of peace and goodness.

So we must be *beholders of the goodness of God.* Become *beholders* of the consistency of his Truth. Be *beholders* of that which has been since before time was. Be *beholders*, not doers. When we react to any circumstance with a sense of urgency, feeling the need to "fix" it, or "rush to do something," we have ceased to be a beholder of what will be revealed to us about our true being. We have not allowed ourselves to see beyond the veil of appearances into the incredible face of God. We have instead danced the dance of doom with the monkeys as they nipped and bit at our legs. We have felt the searing, hot breath of the dragons as they surround us to devour us. We have become a victim to the situation. We have not waited for Wisdom to appear. We have chosen not to be a beholder.

The sense of fear or agitation is actually the doorbell ringing into our souls, demanding entrance. It is an alarm going off saying, "Wait, stop! What is this voice? What are these words that I am listening to? Is this the voice of God, declaring continual goodness? Or is this the voice of man, confused about his identity, believing in his own fears once again?" This is the time to choose. This is the time to know.

If we accept the threats that come as valid, we have ceased to realize that God, the Divine Life of each one of us, is the source of all Life. We have instead believed once again that our bodies are the source of our physical life; our pocketbooks and bank accounts are the source of our security; our relationships are the source of our happiness; and our careers, and positions declare our self worth and determine the stability of our future.

If we instead acknowledge Eternal Life and unchanging Love as the source of our entire existence, we will never *buy into* the appearance of lack or loss again. Right at the moment when the lack or loss is declaring its place and power, we will open our eyes and see through this picture. We will hear the voice of God whispering Its ever-presence to us. We will glorify God as the unhindered, unobstructed, unchanging source of our life and we will see that place filled with the fullness of His truth. We will not declare *how* it will appear, only that it certainly *will*. To declare how something will be resolved is to exercise human will, which always chokes down the flow of Life.

For those of us facing dragons in our life right now, let me paraphrase the first sentence in the popular *Course in Miracles*. There is no order of difficulty in God. The truth is the truth. While it is true that some human fears and beliefs are more frightening and tenacious than others, they still are just that and only that—human beliefs. One moment of looking at reality through the eyes of God, one moment of hearing the slightest suggestion of Truth from His Voice, would dispel whatever the appearance might be, no matter its "order of difficulty." The only thing that matters is that we know that the Source—the original blueprint—NEVER CHANGES.

God is always speaking. Always declaring and revealing the words that will fill and restore any and every human situation. But are we always listening? Do we realize that these words spoken in the secret of our souls are the answers we need to live? Do we know how critical those words are to the peace and success of our life? Have we come to the place where we would rather die, literally, than move a step—before we have heard what step to move? Have we developed, through practice, the courage that it takes to put on the brakes, so to speak, and wait? Have we come to depend on hearing His word of direction, as surely as we depend on our next breath? Or are we still leaning on human solutions, which are so many bondages, and no solutions at all? Are we pausing to *let* the images of Life fill our minds, replacing the images of disease, death and doom? All this will take place as we make a deliberate choice to choose.

We must learn to listen. We "keep the River of Life flowing," not only by our constant attention to love and mercy—which is critical—but also by the moment by moment practice of listening. Joel Goldsmith, in his book *The Thunder of Silence*, describes the voice of God as It roars through the stillness of our souls. Francis Schaeffer wrote a book entitled, *He Is There and He Is Not Silent*. The words fill all space. They are filling every mind and speaking to every heart, every moment of every day. "And thine ears shall hear a word behind thee, saying, This is the way, walk ye in it." (Isaiah)

Today I will be a beholder. I will see beyond the veil of appearances and will behold the wonders of Life. Today I will listen and I will hear and I will know. Today I will behold the wholeness and the completeness that I am. Today I will be a beholder.

CHAPTER TWENTY-SIX

TO BE OUR
OWN HEALER

Life can be lived depending on God alone. He will lead us. He will guide us. He will show us the way. He will never leave us. He will not forsake us. He will impart the understanding necessary for any and every healing. He fills all space. He does not know a vacuum. We are right now walking and talking and living in that space called God. He is as near as our breath. Life was meant to be lived in total reliance on a relationship with our Creator. As such, we will live in perfect harmony. Health and wholeness and peace will be with us daily. We will not fear, even when fear presents itself to us for our attention. This is our inheritance. This is the way it was meant to be. Healing is within our grasp even now. In the silence of our souls, we will know the way. We do not need to scramble around, looking for outside sources of help and relief. They are temporary, at best, and sometimes more destructive than the original problem. Our healing lies within the depths of each one of us. Human struggle is the enemy to total peace. It is the evidence that we do not know Him, Who is our life.

We must look away from our body, for it is but a reflection of the condition of the soul. The affliction that besets us is never the issue, nor the cause, but always the effect. Treating the affliction, the condition of the body alone, is like cutting off diseased branches from a tree. First this branch, then another and another, never dealing with the root cause. We must look away from the affliction; it is only a smoke screen.

Our lives are as a garden and the garden is our soul. We must look to our souls. There we will find the healing that we so desire. We must tend to our souls as we would a cherished garden, watching over it with great love and attention, weeding out the thoughts and daily conflicts that would crowd out the life of it. In the silence of our souls we must allow for peace. When peace fills our being, healing is inevitable, oftentimes instantaneous. Our bodies are a reflection of the condition of our souls. In absolute stillness we realize peace as it flows through our being, bringing life to every part of us.

The only difficulty is reaching that place of quietness. The world will press in for our attention. Our bodies will demand our attention. We must not resist these distractions, nor do we yield to them. We will have to learn to look away, though they seem to be so insistent. Cherish the times of aloneness. Resist the temptation to "fill in the space" with idle nothingness. We do not need to be entertained, every moment filled with activity. Aloneness must not be feared, it is our gift from God. It is the Spirit and Source of all Life knocking on the door of our soul, saying, "Come, be with Me for a moment, and find here the peace and strength and wholeness which is Mine to impart." It is the avenue to total peace and therefore, total restoration. We may realize our healing in a moment of stillness, or it may take many moments of quietness and contemplation. Learn to cherish these times. It is in these times that we develop a deep and lasting and eternal relationship with the source of all peace, and therefore the source of all wholeness. This is where the barriers are removed. This is where the River of Life flows, healing all that it touches. As with anything else we pursue, if we remain constant in this endeavor, if it becomes the most important quest of our life, we will find our life.

> Keep thy heart with all diligence; for out of it are
> the issues of life.
>
> PROVERBS

Suggested Readings and Authors:

The Bible

Andrew Murray — Moody Press, Chicago

E.W. Kenyon — Kenyon's Gospel Publishing Society, Inc. Seattle, Washington

George R. Hawtin — Box 339, Battleford, Sask., Canada, SOM OEO

Hannah Hurnard — *Hinds Feet On High Places*, The Olive Press, 16 Lincoln's Inn Fields, London W.C.2

John Bunyan — *The Pilgrims Progress*, Barbour and Company, Inc. 164 Mill St., Westwood, NJ 07675

Joel Goldsmith — Harper San Francisco - A division of Harper Collins Publishers

Mary Baker Eddy — The First Church of Christ, Scientist, Boston, Mass.

Helen Schucman — *A Course In Miracles*, Penguin Books USA Inc., 375 Hudson St., New York, NY 10014

Marianne Williamson — *A Return To Love*, HarperCollins Publishers, Inc. 10 East 53rd St., New York, NY 10022

Deepak Chopra, M.D., Harmony Books, 201 East 50th St. New York, NY 10022